KU-652-817

Symptoms, Diagnosis and Treatment

A Guide for Pharmacists and Nurses

Paul Rutter BPharm MRPharmS PhD

Senior Lecturer, Pharmacy Practice Division
School of Pharmacy and Biomedical Sciences
University of Portsmouth, UK

GEORGE GREEN LIBRARY OF
SCIENCE AND ENGINEERING

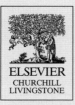

ELSEVIER
CHURCHILL
LIVINGSTONE

Edinburgh London New York Oxford
Philadelphia St Louis Sydney Toronto 2005

ELSEVIER
CHURCHILL
LIVINGSTONE   1005104706

© 2005, Elsevier Limited. All rights reserved.

The right of Paul Rutter to be identified as author of this work has been
asserted by him in accordance with the Copyright, Designs and Patents Act
1988

No part of this publication may be reproduced, stored in a retrieval system, or
transmitted in any form or by any means, electronic, mechanical,
photocopying, recording or otherwise, without either the prior permission of
the publishers or a licence permitting restricted copying in the United
Kingdom issued by the Copyright Licensing Agency, 90 Tottenham Court Road,
London W1T 4LP. Permissions may be sought directly from Elsevier's Health
Sciences Rights Department in Philadelphia, USA: phone: (+1) 215 238 7869,
fax: (+1) 215 238 2239, e-mail: healthpermissions@elsevier.com. You may
also complete your request on-line via the Elsevier homepage
(http://www.elsevier.com), by selecting 'Customer Support' and then
'Obtaining Permissions'.

First published 2005
    Reprinted 2006

ISBN 0 443 07363 5

British Library Cataloguing in Publication Data
A catalogue record for this book is available from the British Library

Library of Congress Cataloguing in Publication Data
A catalogue record for this book is available from the Library of Congress

Notice
Knowledge and best practice in this field are constantly changing. As new
research and experience broaden our knowledge, changes in practice,
treatment and drug therapy may become necessary or appropriate. Readers are
advised to check the most current information provided (i) on procedures
featured or (ii) by the manufacturer of each product to be administered, to
verify the recommended dose or formula, the method and duration of
administration, and contraindications. It is the responsibility of the
practitioner, relying on experience and knowledge of the patient, to make
diagnoses, to determine dosages and the best treatment for each individual
patient, and to take all appropriate safety precautions. To the fullest extent of
the law, neither the publisher nor the authors assumes any liability for any
injury and/or damage.

The Publisher

ELSEVIER   your source for books,
journals and multimedia
in the health sciences
www.elsevierhealth.com

Working together to grow
libraries in developing countries
www.elsevier.com | www.bookaid.org | www.sabre.org
ELSEVIER   BOOK AID International   Sabre Foundation

The
publisher's
policy is to use
**paper manufactured
from sustainable forests**

Printed in China

Contents

Preface

Demand on healthcare professionals to deliver high-quality patient care has never been greater. A multitude of factors impinge on healthcare delivery today, including an ageing population, more sophisticated medicines, high patient expectation, health service funding and staffing levels. In addition there have been massive changes to the structure and organisation of UK health services, especially in primary care. This, coupled with government initiatives and targets, has reinforced the general practitioner's position as the central member of the healthcare team, but at the same time has placed further demands on an already heavy GP workload.

To overcome such problems, the UK government is attempting to implement new models of service delivery by reviewing the way in which other healthcare professionals practise. This is leading to the traditional boundaries of care between doctors, nurses and pharmacists being broken down. GPs and pharmacists have agreed new contracts in 2004 and 2005 which reinforce the collaborative approach to patient care, with service-level agreements encouraging closer working relationships; for example pharmacists to undertake medication reviews and GPs to encourage patients to access community pharmacy services for minor illnesses.

Pharmacists are not the only ones to take on such roles; greater numbers of highly trained nurses are running specialist clinics, e.g. asthma, diabetes or minor illness clinics. These clinics effectively screen and triage patients, thus allowing GPs to concentrate on other patients with multiple or complex problems.

In addition, the government has encouraged manufacturers to make prescription-only medicines more freely available by deregulation to Pharmacy status, allowing pharmacists to treat a growing list of conditions and thus prevent unnecessary GP appointments being made.

Over the next few years deregulation of more medicines looks set to continue and healthcare professionals allied to the GP will have to demonstrate that they are competent practitioners to be trusted with this additional responsibility.

Greater levels of knowledge and understanding about commonly occurring medical conditions will be needed so that they can be recognised and, if appropriate, medication issued using an evidence-based approach to treatment.

This is the catalyst for this book. Although other books on diagnosis are available to pharmacists and nurses, this book aims to give a practical primary care perspective on minor conditions.

It is hoped that the information contained within the book is both informative and useful.

Paul Rutter

Introduction

Communication skills

In general, most pharmacists and, to a lesser extent, nurses will be dependent on their ability to question patients in order to arrive at a differential diagnosis. This is in stark contrast to the GP, who routinely draws on physical examination and diagnostic tests to help arrive at a diagnosis. Despite this, a number of studies have shown that the correct diagnosis can be achieved in three-quarters of all cases by taking a patient history alone.

It is therefore extremely important that nurses and pharmacists possess excellent communication skills to ensure that the correct information is obtained from the patient. This will be drawn from a combination of good questioning technique, listening actively to the patient and picking up on non-verbal cues.

Approaches to differential diagnosis

A number of methods can be employed to gain information from the patient to arrive at a differential diagnosis. Acronyms can be used to act as prompts to allow the healthcare practitioner to remember what questions to ask but are often inadequate as they are rigid and inflexible. Asking questions from a harm minimisation approach is another method. This technique tends to be used by NHS Direct; sinister pathology is first ruled out before asking questions on more likely conditions that the person will be suffering from. This second approach, in a primary care setting, can be time-consuming and impractical. A method often advocated in medical undergraduate training is diagnostic reasoning or clinical decision making.

Clinical decision making

Whether we are conscious of it or not, most people will – at some level – use clinical decision making to arrive at a differential diagnosis. Diagnostic reasoning is a component of clinical decision making and involves recognition of cues and analysis of data. Very early in a clinical encounter, and based on limited information, a practitioner will arrive at a small number of hypotheses. The practitioner then sets about testing these hypotheses by asking the patient a series of questions. The answer to each question allows the practitioner to narrow down the possible diagnosis either by eliminating particular conditions or by confirming his or her suspicions of a particular condition. Once questioning is over, the practitioner should be in a position to differentially diagnose the patient's condition.

Key steps in the process

1. Formulating a diagnosis based on the patient and the initial presenting complaint

Before any questions are asked of the patient you should already begin to be thinking about the line of questioning you are going to take.

- What is the general appearance of the patient? Does the person look well or poorly? Is the person you are about to talk to the patient or someone acting on the patient's behalf? This will shape your thinking as to the severity of the problem.
- How old is the patient? This is very useful information. Epidemiological studies for a wide range of conditions and disease states have shown that certain age groups will suffer from certain problems. For example, it is very unlikely that a child who presents with cough will have chronic bronchitis, but the probability of an elderly person having chronic bronchitis is much higher.
- What sex is the patient? As with age, sex can dramatically alter the chances of suffering from certain conditions. Migraines are five times more common in women than in men, yet cluster headache is nine times more common in men than in women.
- What is the presenting complaint? Some conditions are much more common than others. Therefore, you could form an idea of what condition the patient is likely to be suffering from based on the laws of probability. For example, if a person presents with a headache then you should already know that the most common cause of headache

is tension headache, followed by migraine and then cluster headache. Other causes of headache are rare but obviously need to be eliminated. Your line of questioning should try to confirm or refute the most likely causes of headache.

2. Asking questions

The questions you ask the patient will be specific to that patient. After establishing who the person is, how poorly he or she is and what the presenting complaint is, a number of targeted questions specific to that patient should be asked. The following scenario will illustrate this point:

A 31-year-old female asks for advice about a headache she has. What are your initial thoughts? (1. Formulating a diagnosis based on the patient and the initial presenting complaint):

- the patient is present
- the patient is female and in her early 30s
- the patient looks and sounds OK
- epidemiology states that tension headache is most likely but females are more prone to migraine than males.

What line of questioning do you take? (2. Asking questions). Your main aim is to differentiate between tension and migraine headache:

Nature of the pain
Tension headache usually produces a dull ache, as opposed to the throbbing nature of migraine pain:

- patient's response: dull ache
- practitioner's thoughts: suggestive of tension headache.

Location of the pain
Tension headache is generally bilateral; migraine is often unilateral:

- patient's response: all over
- practitioner's thoughts: suggestive of tension headache.

Severity of the pain
Tension headache is not usually severe and disabling; migraine can be disabling:

- patient's response: bothersome more than stopping her doing things
- practitioner's thoughts: suggestive of tension headache.

The answers so far are indicative of tension headache. However, further specific questions relating to lifestyle and previous and family history should be asked. It would be expected that there was no family history of migraine and there is probably some trigger factor causing the headache, for example increased stress due to work or personal pressures. The patient might therefore have had similar headaches in the past.

Finally, even though at this stage you are confident of your differential diagnosis you should still ask a couple of questions to rule out any sinister pathology. Obviously, you are expecting the answers from these questions to be negative to support your differential diagnosis. Any questions that invoke the opposite response to that expected will require further investigation.

3. Confirm facts

Before making a recommendation to the patient it is always helpful to try and recap on the information elicited. This is especially important when you have had to ask a lot of questions. It is well known that short-term working memory is relatively small and that remembering all the pertinent facts is difficult. Summarising the information at this stage will not only help you formulate your final diagnosis but will also allow the patient to add further information or to correct you on facts that you have failed to remember correctly.

The way in which one goes about establishing what is wrong with the patient will vary from practitioner to practitioner. However, it is important that whatever method is adopted must be sufficiently robust to be of benefit to the patient. Using a clinical decision-making approach to differential diagnosis allows you to build a fuller picture of the patient's presenting complaint. It is both flexible and specific to each individual, unlike acronyms.

How to use this book

This book is divided into 10 chapters. The first nine are systems based and structured in the format shown in Fig. 1. The final chapter is product based and has a slightly different format.

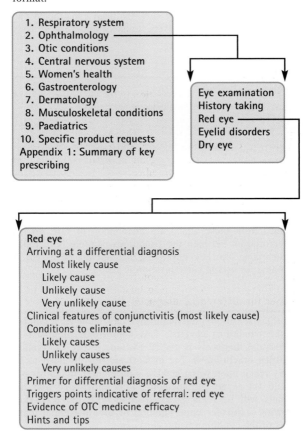

1. Respiratory system
2. Ophthalmology
3. Otic conditions
4. Central nervous system
5. Women's health
6. Gastroenterology
7. Dermatology
8. Musculoskeletal conditions
9. Paediatrics
10. Specific product requests
Appendix 1: Summary of key prescribing

Eye examination
History taking
Red eye
Eyelid disorders
Dry eye

Red eye
Arriving at a differential diagnosis
    Most likely cause
    Likely cause
    Unlikely cause
    Very unlikely cause
Clinical features of conjunctivitis (most likely cause)
Conditions to eliminate
    Likely causes
    Unlikely causes
    Very unlikely causes
Primer for differential diagnosis of red eye
Triggers points indicative of referral: red eye
Evidence of OTC medicine efficacy
Hints and tips

Key features of each chapter

For each condition the same structure has been adopted. This is intended to help the reader approach differential diagnosis from the position of clinical decision making. To help summarise some of the information, tables and algorithms are included for many of the conditions.

Arriving at a differential diagnosis

For each condition, e.g. red eye, a list of possible conditions most often seen in primary care has been constructed and divided into most likely, likely, unlikely and very unlikely causes.

Probability	Cause
Most likely	Bacterial or allergic conjunctivitis
Likely	Viral conjunctivitis, subconjunctival haemorrhage
Unlikely	Episcleritis, scleritis, keratitis, uveitis
Very unlikely	Acute closed-angle glaucoma

This enables the reader to quickly differentiate those conditions that are common (as shown from epidemiological studies) from those which are uncommon or rare. To aid differentiation between the conditions, a table is included summarising the key questions that should be asked. A rationale for asking each question is stated.

Primer for differential diagnosis

A 'primer for differential diagnosis' is available for a number of the conditions covered. This algorithmic approach to differential diagnosis is geared towards nearly or recently qualified practitioners. The primers are not intended to be solely relied upon when making a differential diagnosis but should act as an aide-memoire. It is anticipated that the primers will be used in conjunction with the text, thus allowing a broader understanding of the differential diagnosis of the condition being considered.

Triggers points indicative of referral

A summary box of trigger factors when it would be prudent to refer the patient to a medical practitioner is presented for each condition.

Evidence of OTC medicine efficacy

This section presents the reader with an evaluation of the current literature on whether the over-the-counter medicine works. Trial data, where available, have been reviewed and each product's effectiveness assessed. In the Appendix, product choice is differentiated into first and second line options based on the evidence.

Hints and tips

A summary box of useful information is provided near the end of each condition. This contains information that does not fall readily into any of the other sections but is none the less useful. For example, prolonged use of ocular vaso-constrictors can cause rebound redness on withdrawal of the medication.

Appendix: practical prescribing

For the products reviewed, practical prescribing information is given and separated into:

- condition, alphabetically listed
- treatment
  - first line
  - second line
- dosing
- likely side-effects
- significant drug interactions
- care needed (and includes)
  - pregnancy and breast-feeding
  - liver disease
  - renal impairment.

This appendix is meant to act as a quick reference but does not replace standard textbooks such as *Stockley's Drug Interactions*, Briggs' *Drugs in Pregnancy and Lactation* or manufacturers' summaries of product characteristics, which will give fuller and more comprehensive information.

Finally, all information presented in the book is accurate and factual as far as the author is aware. It is acknowledged that guidelines change, products become discontinued and new information becomes available over the lifetime of a book. Therefore, if any information in the book is not current or valid, the author would be grateful of any feedback, positive or negative, to ensure that the next edition is as up to date as possible.

Chapter 1

Respiratory system

Respiratory conditions are one of the most common problems encountered by primary care practitioners. Conditions such as cough, cold and sore throat are extremely common, with the average GP seeing between 700 and 1000 patients with respiratory disease each year.

Cough

The main function of coughing is airway clearance. Coughs can be described as productive (chesty) or non-productive (dry, tight, tickly). Many patients will deny that they are producing sputum but might say that they 'can feel it on their chest'. In these cases the cough is probably productive and should be treated as such. Coughs can be classed as acute (< 3 weeks' duration) or chronic (> 3 weeks). Chronic coughs should be referred to a medical practitioner.

Arriving at a differential diagnosis

The most likely cause of acute cough in primary care for all ages is viral infection. Practitioners should therefore direct questions to confirm this diagnosis as other conditions can give rise to symptoms of cough and are listed below.

Probability	Cause
Most likely	Viral infection
Likely	Postnasal drip, allergy
Unlikely	Croup, chronic bronchitis, asthma, pneumonia, ACE inhibitor
Very unlikely	Heart failure, bronchiectasis, tuberculosis, cancer, pneumothorax, lung abscess, nocardiasis, GORD

ACE, angiotensin-converting enzyme; GORD, gastro-oesophageal reflux disease.

Clinical features of acute viral cough

Viral coughs typically present with sudden onset, fever and associated cold symptoms. Sputum production is minimal and symptoms are often worse in the evening. These coughs usually last 7–10 days. A number of other factors need to be considered, e.g. when the cough occurs and previous and medical history to ensure that the assumption of viral cough is correct. Table 1.1 lists the questions that should be asked to help determine the diagnosis.

Table 1.1
Specific questions to ask the patient: cough

Question	Relevance

Sputum colour	• Mucoid (clear and white), yellow/green/brown sputum suggests viral infection.
	• Haemoptysis suggests sinister pathology: **refer**
	  – Rust-coloured sputum suggests pneumonia
	  – Pink-tinged sputum suggests left ventricular failure
	  – Dark-red sputum suggests carcinoma

Nature of sputum	• Thin and frothy suggests left ventricular failure: **refer** • Thick/mucoid suggests asthma • Offensive, foul-smelling sputum suggests bronchiectasis or lung abscess: **refer**
Onset of cough	• Worse in the morning suggests postnasal drip, bronchiectasis or chronic bronchitis • If a child has a non-productive cough at night this suggests asthma

Duration of cough	• >1 week and mucopurulent sputum suggests bacterial infection
	• The longer the duration the more likely underlying pathology is responsible:
	  – Cough of 3 days suggests viral infection
	  – Cough of 3 weeks suggests acute or chronic bronchitis
	  – Cough of 3 months suggests chronic bronchitis, tuberculosis or carcinoma

Question	Relevance
Periodicity	● In adults, especially if they smoke, recurrent cough suggests chronic bronchitis ● In children, a recurrent cough and family history of eczema, asthma or hay fever suggest asthma
Age of the patient	● Cough in children suggests an upper respiratory tract infection ● In a child a non-productive cough at night suggests asthma ● Increasing age increases the chances of more sinister pathology, e.g. bronchitis, pneumonia and carcinoma
Smoking history	● Smokers are more prone to chronic and recurrent cough. Over time this could develop into chronic bronchitis and emphysema

Conditions to eliminate

Likely causes

Postnasal drip This is characterised by sinus or nasal discharge that flows in to the throat. Patients should be asked if they are swallowing mucus or clearing their throat more than usual, as these are common symptoms in patients with postnasal drip.

Allergy-related cough Cough is non-productive and often worse at night. Other associated symptoms are usually present, e.g. sneezing, nasal discharge/blockage and conjunctivitis. Cough of allergic origin might show seasonal variation, e.g. hay fever.

Unlikely causes

Laryngotracheobronchitis (croup) Croup primarily affects infants aged 9–18 months. The cough is described as having a barking quality and often occurs after an upper respiratory tract infection. Attacks typically occur in the middle of the night and subside within a few hours.

Chronic bronchitis (CB) This is the most common cause of chronic cough in adults. Patients usually present with a longstanding history of recurrent acute bronchitis. A history of smoking is the single most important factor in the aetiology of chronic bronchitis. Cough is normally productive.

Asthma Asthma is characterised by coughing, wheeze, chest tightness and shortness of breath. However, asthma can present solely as a non-productive cough. This is especially true in young children, in whom the cough often worsens at night.

Pneumonia Initially, the cough is non-productive and painful but it rapidly becomes productive, with sputum being stained red. The cough tends to worsen at night. The patient will be unwell and suffer from a high fever, malaise, chills, headache and pleuritic pain.

Medicine-induced cough or wheeze Angiotensin-converting enzyme (ACE) inhibitors are most commonly associated with cough and can affect up to one in five patients.

Very unlikely causes

Heart failure Heart failure is a condition of the elderly. It is characterised by insidious progression, the first symptoms being shortness of breath and dyspnoea at night. As the condition progresses the patient might develop a productive, frothy cough, which may be pink tinged.

Bronchiectasis Characteristically, the patient has a chronic cough of very long duration that produces copious amounts of mucopurulent sputum that is usually foul smelling.

Tuberculosis (TB) Tuberculosis is characterised by its slow onset and initial mild symptoms. The cough is chronic in nature and sputum production can vary from mild to severe with associated haemoptysis. Other symptoms of the condition are malaise, fever, night sweats and weight loss.

Carcinoma of the lung Lung cancer is associated with long-term cigarette smokers who have had a cough for a number of months or who develop a marked change in the character of their cough. The cough produces small amounts of sputum, which might be blood streaked. Dyspnoea, weight loss and fatigue might also be seen.

Spontaneous pneumothorax (collapsed lung)   This most frequently affects tall, thin men aged 20–40 years. The patient experiences sudden sharp chest pain that worsens on chest movement. Smoking and a family history of pneumothorax are contributing risk factors.

Lung abscess   A typical presentation is of a non-productive cough with pleuritic pain, dyspnoea, malaise and fever. In time the cough produces large amounts of purulent and often foul-smelling sputum.

Nocardiosis   There is a productive cough producing purulent, thick and possibly blood-tinged sputum. Fever is prominent and night sweats, pleurisy, weight loss and fatigue might also be present.

Gastro–oesophageal reflux disease (GORD)   Reflux does not usually present with cough, but patients with this condition may cough when lying down. It should always be considered in all cases of unexplained chronic cough.

Primer for differential diagnosis

Figure 1.1 helps to differentiate between serious and non-serious conditions of cough.

TRIGGER POINTS indicative of referral: cough

- Chest pain.
- Chronic cough (> 3 weeks).
- Cough that recurs on a regular basis.
- Haemoptysis.
- Pain on inspiration.
- Persistent nocturnal cough in children.
- Wheeze and/or shortness of breath.

Evidence of OTC medicine efficacy

Efficacy trials involving cough medicines are limited. They suffer from poor design and low patient numbers and have

Figure 1.1 Primer for differential diagnosis of cough in adults.

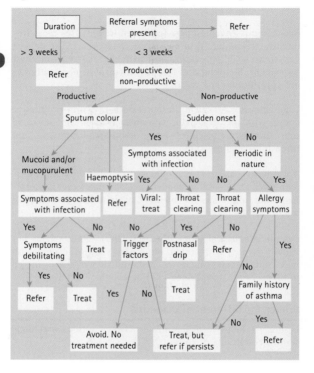

often been conducted in animals or healthy volunteers. Clinical evidence of efficacy is therefore difficult to establish. However, a systematic review of OTC cough medicines (expectorants, antihistamines and antitussives) for acute coughs in adults was published in the *British Medical Journal* in 2002. Fifteen trials involving 2166 participants/ patients met the authors' inclusion criteria. In nine of the trials the active ingredient was no better than placebo and the authors of the review questioned the clinical relevance of the other six trials that showed positive findings. In conclusion, the authors stated that OTC cough medicines for acute cough cannot be recommended because there is no good evidence of effectiveness.

HINTS AND TIPS

- Avoid theophylline products: theophylline can help with wheeze or shortness of breath and is available OTC. However, such symptoms should be referred to the GP.
- Avoid illogical combinations: there are still a few products on the market that have illogical cough ingredient combinations, e.g. combinations of expectorants and suppressants (Pulmo Bailey) or expectorant and antihistamines (e.g. Histalix).
- Coughs lasting longer than 3 weeks: most acute, self-limiting coughs resolve within 3 weeks. However, not all coughs that have lasted 3 weeks have to be referred automatically. Postnasal drip and seasonal allergies (e.g. hay fever) can persist for weeks.

Cough medication for children

Very few well-designed studies have been conducted in children. It appears from the limited data that cough medication for children is no better than placebo.

Practical prescribing

Prescribing information relating to cough medication is summarised in the appendix.

The common cold

Colds, along with coughs, represent the largest caseload for primary healthcare workers. Depending on age, people suffer 3–12 colds per year.

Arriving at a differential diagnosis

The most likely cause of cold symptoms in primary care for all ages is a viral infection. Practitioners should therefore direct questions to confirm this diagnosis as other conditions can give rise to cold symptoms and are listed below.

Probability	Cause
Most likely	Viral infection
Likely	Seasonal allergic rhinitis (hay fever), sinusitis
Unlikely	Influenza, perennial rhinitis

Clinical features of the common cold

Symptoms of the common cold are well known. Usually, symptoms start with sore throat and sneezing followed by nasal discharge/congestion. Cough and postnasal drip commonly follow, often accompanied by headache, fever and general malaise. Common colds can last for 14 days or more.

Table 1.2 lists some of the questions that should be asked to aid diagnosis.

Conditions to eliminate

Likely causes

Seasonal allergic rhinitis (hay fever)   Patients experience a combination of or all four classic rhinitis symptoms of nasal itch, sneeze, rhinorrhoea and nasal congestion. Hay fever sufferers also commonly experience allergic conjunctivitis and experience symptoms from March to October.

Acute sinusitis   Acute sinusitis is a complication of the common cold. Pain in the early stages is relatively localised, usually unilateral and dull but might become bilateral and more severe the longer the condition persists. Bending down, coughing or sneezing often exacerbates the pain. If the ethmoid sinuses (located near to and behind the bridge of the nose) are involved then pain behind the eye(s) is often experienced.

Otitis media   Most common in children, otitis media presents as ear pain, accompanied by fever often after or during a cold. Pain is relieved once the eardrum ruptures causing purulent discharge, which usually lasts 2–3 days.

Table 1.2
Specific questions to ask the patient: the common cold

Question	Relevance
Onset of symptoms	• Flu is normally seen in the winter months whereas the common cold can occur at any time • Flu symptoms tend to be more abrupt in onset than the common cold, starting in hours rather than 1 or 2 days • Summer colds are common but they must be differentiated from seasonal allergic rhinitis (hay fever)
Nature of symptoms	• Marked myalgia, chills and malaise are more prominent in flu than the common cold. Loss of appetite is also common with flu
Aggravating factors	• If headache/pain is worsened when sneezing, coughing and bending over, this suggests sinus complications • If ear pain is present, especially in children, this suggests middle ear involvement

Unlikely causes

Influenza Flu symptoms present in a similar fashion to those of the common cold but are usually more severe. Patients with flu are likely to be bed-bound and debilitated. A patient who presents to a healthcare professional claiming to have flu is much more likely to have a cold.

TRIGGER POINTS indicative of referral: cold

- Acute sinus involvement.
- Ear pain originating from the middle ear.
- Patients with symptoms indicative of flu.
- Vulnerable patient groups, such as the very elderly.

Evidence of OTC medicine efficacy

Many of the active ingredients found in cold remedies are also constituents of cough products. In many cases they are combined and marketed as cough/cold or flu remedies.

Antihistamines

A review article published in the *Journal of the American Medical Association* in 1993 on OTC cold medications concluded that only chlorphenamine reduced sneezing and decreased symptom scores. Other antihistamines (diphenhydramine and triprolidine) were no better than placebo.

Systemic and topical sympathomimetics

Sympathomimetics are clinically effective, although only pseudoephedrine (systemic) and oxymetazoline (topical) have trial data to support their efficacy.

Multi-ingredient preparations

No multi-ingredient preparation has specific trial data to substantiate its effectiveness, but they often contain ingredients that have known clinical efficacy, e.g. decongestants and analgesia. In the majority of cases patients will not require all the active ingredients within the preparation to treat their symptoms. A more sensible approach to treatment is to match symptoms with active ingredients with known efficacy. This can be achieved in many cases by providing the patient with monotherapy or a product containing two active ingredients.

Alternative therapies

Many products are advocated to help treat cold symptoms, in particular zinc, vitamin C and echinacea.

Zinc lozenges
There is a growing body of evidence to show that zinc can decrease the duration and severity of the common cold, although the evidence is based on small studies.

Vitamin C
Vitamin C has been widely recommended as a 'cure' for the common cold, but whether or not it is effective remains con-

troversial. Recent large-scale reviews (Douglas et al, Cochrane Library issue 3, 2004) of trial data have concluded that vitamin C does not prevent colds but may reduce the duration of cold symptoms when ingested in high doses (up to 1 g daily).

Echinacea

Current evidence is conflicting. Some studies suggest that echinacea preparations might be better than placebo at decreasing the duration of the common cold, but there is no strong evidence to recommend a specific echinacea product or dosage. Other studies have shown no effect (e.g. Yale et al, *Arch Intern Med* 2004; 164: 1237–1241).

Steam inhalation

Current trial data support the use of vapour inhalation in relieving the symptoms of the common cold. It appears that steam is the key to symptom resolution and not any additional ingredients that might be added to the water.

Practical prescribing

Prescribing information relating to cold medication is summarised in the appendix.

HINTS AND TIPS

- Stuffy noses in babies: saline nose drops can be used from birth to help with congestion.
- General sales list (GSL) cold remedies: products such as the Lemsip and Beechams range contain paracetamol. It is important to ensure patients are not taking excessive doses of analgesia unknowingly. Also, many contain subtherapeutic doses of sympathomimetics. If a sympathomimetic is needed then these products are best avoided.
- Administration of nose drops: the best way to administer nose drops is to have the head in the downwards position facing the floor. Tilting the head backwards and towards the ceiling is incorrect as it facilitates the swallowing of the drops. However, most patients will find the latter way of putting drops in to the nose much easier than the former.

Sore throat

Most adults experience two or three sore throats each year. Symptoms can range from mild to severe pain.

Arriving at a differential diagnosis

The most likely cause of sore throat in primary care for all ages is a viral infection. Practitioners should therefore direct questions to confirm this diagnosis as other conditions can give rise to sore throat and are listed below.

Probability	Cause
Most likely	Viral infection
Likely	Streptococcal infection
Unlikely	Thrush, herpes simplex, glandular fever, trauma
Very unlikely	Carcinoma, medicines

Clinical features of viral sore throat

Sore throat is the most obvious symptom but there might be other systemic symptoms such as malaise, fever, headache and cough. Symptoms spontaneously resolve after about 7–10 days.

Differentiation between viral and other causes of sore throat must be made before treatment is given. Table 1.3 lists a number of questions that should be asked to help diagnosis.

Physical examination

After questioning, an inspection of the mouth should be performed. Use a good light source (e.g. pen torch). Ask the patient to open the mouth and to say 'ah'; this should allow you to see the pharynx well. When examining the mouth pay particular attention to the fauces and tonsils. Are they red and swollen? Is any exudate present? Is there any sign of ulceration? Also feel the cervical glands (located just below the angle of the jaw) to see if they are swollen.

Table 1.3
Specific questions to ask the patient: sore throat

Question	Relevance
Age of the patient	● Streptococcal infections are more prevalent in school-aged children ● Glandular fever is most prevalent in adolescents ● Oral thrush affects the very young and very old
Tender cervical glands	● Marked swollen glands suggest glandular fever or streptococcal sore throat. This is less so in viral sore throat
Tonsillar exudate present	● Marked tonsillar exudate suggests a bacterial cause
Nature of the pain	● True difficulty in swallowing (not just pain when swallowing) suggests a mechanical blockage (e.g. carcinoma): **refer**

Conditions to eliminate

Likely causes

Streptococcal sore throat A sore throat that has lasted longer than 1 week can suggest a streptococcal infection, especially if accompanied by marked tonsillar exudate, tender cervical glands, a temperature of over 101°F (39.4°C) and the absence of cough.

Unlikely causes

Glandular fever (infectious mononucleosis) Patients with glandular fever are typically adolescents and young adults. Symptoms are characterised by pharyngitis, fever, cervical lymphadenopathy and fatigue. The person might also have suffered from general malaise prior to the onset of the other symptoms.

Sore throat caused by trauma Occasionally patients develop a sore throat from direct irritation of the pharynx. This might be due to cigarette smoke, a lodged foreign body or acid reflux.

Oral thrush Pain and soreness is often present but in oral thrush soft, elevated, creamy-white patches anywhere in the oral cavity should be present.

Herpes simplex infection This is a common cause of oral ulceration in children. Primary infection results in ulceration of the gums, tongue and cheeks but can affect any part of the oral mucosa, leading to sore throat. Multiple ulcers should be visible on examination. The infection spontaneously resolves in 7–14 days.

Very unlikely causes

Medicine-induced sore throat Agranulocytosis (decrease in all white blood cells) is associated with a number of medicines:

- captopril
- carbimazole
- cytotoxics
- neuroleptics, e.g. clozapine
- penicillamine
- sulfasalazine
- sulphur-containing antibiotics.

Laryngeal and tonsillar carcinoma Both these cancers have a strong link with smoking and excessive alcohol intake, and are more common in men than in women. Sore throat and dysphagia are the common presenting symptoms. Patients with tonsillar cancer often develop referred ear pain.

TRIGGER POINTS indicative of referral: sore throat

- Adverse drug reaction.
- Associated skin rash.
- Duration > 2 weeks.
- Dysphagia.
- Marked tonsillar exudate accompanied by a high temperature and swollen glands.

Primer for differential diagnosis of sore throat

Figure 1.2 helps to differentiate between serious and non-serious conditions in which sore throat is a major presenting complaint.

15

Evidence of OTC medicine efficacy

OTC medication is either topical, containing antibacterials and anaesthetics, or systemic analgesia.

Figure 1.2   Primer for differential diagnosis of sore throat.

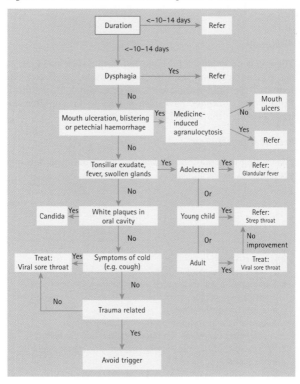

16

Local anaesthetics (lidocaine and benzocaine)

Very few trials involving products marketed for sore throat have been conducted, and it appears that manufacturers are using trial data on local anaesthetic efficacy for conditions other than sore throats to substantiate their effect.

Antibacterial and antifungal agents

These products should not be routinely recommended because viruses cause most sore throats and these agents have no action against viruses.

Anti-inflammatories

Benzydamine is available as a spray or mouthwash and has proven efficacy in relieving the pain associated with sore throat.

Analgesia

There is good evidence to show that simple systemic analgesia, e.g. paracetamol, aspirin and ibuprofen, is effective in reducing the pain associated with sore throat. In addition, flurbiprofen lozenges have also shown to be significantly more effective than placebo in reducing pain.

Practical prescribing

Prescribing information relating to sore throat medication is summarised in the appendix.

HINTS AND TIPS

- Stimulation of saliva production: sucking a lozenge or pastille promotes saliva production, which will lubricate the throat and exert a soothing action.
- Anaesthetic preparations: pastilles containing local anaesthetics can numb the tongue rather than the throat. Sprays which direct the anaesthetic onto the throat might be more useful.

Allergic rhinitis

Allergic rhinitis is either seasonal (hay fever) or year round (perennial rhinitis) and characterised by rhinorrhoea, nasal congestion, sneezing and itching. It is becoming more common, with the prevalence doubling in the last 30 years.

Arriving at a differential diagnosis

The most likely cause of allergic rhinitis encountered in primary care is hay fever. Practitioners should therefore direct questions to confirm this diagnosis as other conditions cause rhinitis and are listed below.

Probability	Cause
Most likely	Hay fever
Likely	Viral infection, perennial rhinitis
Unlikely	Vasomotor rhinitis, pregnancy, medicines, nasal foreign bodies, polyps

Clinical features of hay fever

The patient will experience a combination of nasal itch, sneeze, rhinorrhoea and nasal congestion, and in addition might have conjunctivitis. Symptoms occur intermittently (i.e. at times of pollen exposure) and tend to be worse in the morning/evening or when the weather is hot and humid. Diagnosis is largely dependent on the patient having a family history of atopy and clinical symptoms. Table 1.4 lists the questions that should be asked to help determine the cause.

Conditions to eliminate

Likely causes

Infective rhinitis Infective rhinitis is associated with the common cold. Nasal discharge tends to be more mucopurulent than allergic rhinitis and nasal itching is uncommon. Sneezing tends not to occur in paroxysms and symptoms usually resolve within a couple of weeks. This in contrast to allergic rhinitis, which lasts for as long as the person is

Table 1.4
Specific questions to ask the patient: rhinitis

Question	Relevance
Timing	● Symptoms in the summer months suggest hay fever ● Year-round symptoms suggest perennial rhinitis
History of atopy in the family	● If a parent suffers from atopy then hay fever is the most likely cause of rhinitis in children
Effect of pollen	● Pollen is the main allergen in hay fever. When pollen counts are high, symptoms will worsen ● Infective rhinitis will be unaffected by pollen count ● Patients with perennial rhinitis can suffer from worsening symptoms but symptoms will still persist when unexposed to pollen (e.g. indoors) because house-dust mite and animal dander are the main allergens

exposed to the allergen. Other symptoms, such as cough and sore throat, are much more prominent in infective rhinitis.

Perennial allergic rhinitis Perennial allergic rhinitis is 10 times less common than hay fever. Symptoms tend to be experienced year-round but may worsen in the summer months. Nasal congestion is common and patients are more prone to sinusitis. The sense of smell can be diminished and patients tend to suffer from less sneezing and conjunctivitis than those with hay fever.

Unlikely causes

Vasomotor rhinitis Symptoms are very similar to allergic rhinitis yet an allergy test will be negative. Itching and sneezing are less common and patients may experience worsening nasal symptoms in response to climactic factors such as a sudden change in temperature.

Rhinitis of pregnancy   This occurs due to hormonal changes and resolves spontaneously after childbirth.

Rhinitis medicamentosa   Prolonged use of topical decongestants can cause rebound vasodilatation of the nasal arterioles leading to further nasal congestion. A medication history should be taken from the patient.

Nasal blockage or foreign body   If congestion is the only symptom, it is possible that the problem is mechanical or anatomical. Continuous and unilateral blockage might relate to a deviated nasal septum in adults or a trapped foreign body in young children. Bilateral obstruction might relate to nasal polyps in adults.

Primer for differential diagnosis

Figure 1.3 helps to aid differentiation of the different types of rhinitis.

TRIGGER POINTS indicative of referral: rhinitis

- Failed medication.
- Medicine-induced rhinitis.
- Nasal obstruction that fails to clear.
- Unilateral discharge, especially in children.

Evidence of OTC medicine efficacy

Allergen avoidance

Avoidance of pollen is almost impossible but exposure can be diminished, e.g. staying indoors when pollen counts are high, keeping windows closed and wearing 'wrap around' sunglasses. House-dust mite and animal dander are more easily avoided. The offending pet can be kept out of certain parts of the house, such as living areas and bedrooms. Using allergen-impermeable bed linen and acaricidal sprays can reduce house-dust mite. Replacing carpeted rooms with wooden flooring will also help reduce both animal dander and house-dust mite.

Figure 1.3 Primer for differential diagnosis of rhinitis.

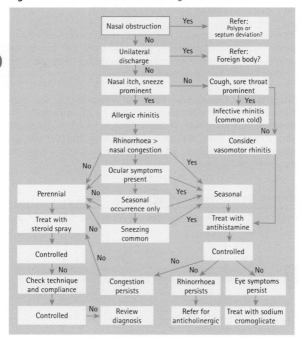

Medication (systemic or topical)

Systemic therapy

Both sedating and non-sedating antihistamines have proven efficacy but, given the sedative properties of older sedating antihistamines, these should not be routinely recommended; however, it is not true that non-sedating antihistamines never cause sedation. A review in the *British Medical Journal* (2000) showed that loratadine causes the least sedation of all antihistamines and, on this basis, would be the antihistamine of choice.

Topical therapy (intranasal or intraocular)

Corticosteroids are the medicine of choice when nasal congestion is the major symptom. WHO recommendations and a meta-analysis (Weiner et al, *Br Med J* 1998; 317:

1624–1629) have concluded that corticosteroids are superior to systemic antihistamines. Other topical agents with proven efficacy include antihistamines (azelastine and levocabastine) and decongestants (although only oxymetazoline appears to have trial data to support its efficacy). Evidence of efficacy via the nasal route is least for sodium cromoglicate.

Intraocular medication

Trials have shown sodium cromoglicate and the antihistamine levocabastine to be superior to placebo and equally effective. Sympathomimetics (e.g. naphazoline) do decrease ocular redness but can cause rebound redness with prolonged use, so, if used, they should be restricted to short-term use. A combination antihistamine/decongestant product is also available (Otrivine Antistin) but there are few trial data to support its effectiveness; one small trial concluded that the combination of the two drugs was superior to either alone (Abelson et al, *Am J Ophthalmol* 1980; 90: 254–257).

Practical prescribing

Prescribing information relating to rhinitis medication is summarised in the appendix.

HINTS AND TIPS

- Corticosteroid nasal sprays: for full therapeutic benefit, regular use is essential. The patient should also be warned that maximum relief might not be obtained for several days.
- Breakthrough symptoms with one-a-day antihistamines: patients who suffer breakthrough symptoms using a once-daily preparation (loratadine, cetirizine) might benefit from changing to acrivastine as three-times-a-day dosing might confer better symptom control.

Chapter 2

Ophthalmology

The main role of primary healthcare professionals is to differentiate between conditions that are minor and self-limiting and those that are serious and sight-threatening. It is therefore important to be able to take an eye history and to perform a simple eye examination.

The eye examination

A great deal of information can be learned from a close inspection of the eye. You can check the size of the pupils, their comparative size and reaction to light, the colour of the sclera, the nature of any discharge and if the eyelid is involved.

The eye should be examined in good light. The basic steps to perform a simple eye examination are as follows:

1. Wash your hands.
2. Ask the patient to sit down and look straight ahead.
3. Gently pull down the lower lid and ask the patient to look upwards and to both the left and the right; this allows the conjunctiva to be examined.
4. Using a pen torch check the reaction of the pupils to light. Shine the light briefly onto the eye and look for constriction of the pupil. Any abnormal pupil reaction should be referred.
5. Check visual acuity by asking the patient to read small print with the affected eye.
6. Wash your hands.

History taking

A number of questions should be asked. Check the severity of pain experienced, the nature of the discharge (if present) and if there is a family history for eye disease (e.g. glaucoma). Also take a current medication history.

Red eye

Redness of the eye and inflammation of the conjunctiva (conjunctivitis) is very common. The exact prevalence of conjunctivitis is not known, although the prevalence of seasonal allergic conjunctivitis (hay fever) is increasing.

Arriving at a differential diagnosis

24

The most likely cause of red eye in primary care is some form of conjunctivitis. Practitioners should therefore direct questions to confirm this diagnosis as other conditions can cause red eye and are listed below.

Probability	Cause
Most likely	Bacterial or allergic conjunctivitis
Likely	Viral conjunctivitis, subconjunctival haemorrhage
Unlikely	Episcleritis, scleritis, keratitis, uveitis
Very unlikely	Acute closed-angle glaucoma

Clinical features of conjunctivitis

Irrespective of the cause – bacterial (Fig. 2.1), allergic (Fig. 2.2) or viral (Fig. 2.3) – conjunctivitis presents similarly with symptoms of redness, discharge and discomfort. Table 2.1 acts as a quick reference to aid differentiation between the different forms.

Table 2.2 highlights questions that should be asked to help confirm the diagnosis of conjunctivitis and rule out more sinister pathology.

Conditions to eliminate

Likely causes

Subconjunctival haemorrhage   A segment of eye, or sometimes the whole eye, will appear bright red (Fig. 2.4); there is no pain. It occurs spontaneously but can be precipitated by coughing, straining or lifting. Symptoms will resolve in 10–14 days without treatment.

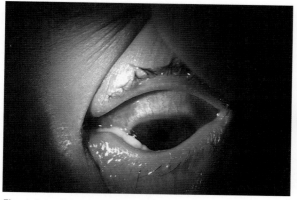

Figure 2.1 Bacterial conjunctivitis. Reproduced from *Handbook of Ocular Disease Management* by Joseph W Sowka OD, Andrew S Gurwood OD and Alan Kabat OD, Jobson Publishing, with permission.

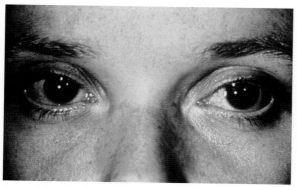

Figure 2.2 Allergic conjunctivitis. Reproduced from *Handbook of Ocular Disease Management* by Joseph W Sowka OD, Andrew S Gurwood OD and Alan Kabat OD, Jobson Publishing, with permission.

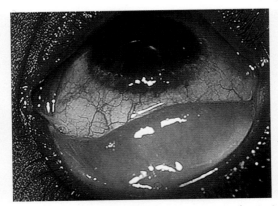

Figure 2.3 Viral conjunctivitis. Reproduced from *Handbook of Ocular Disease Management* by Joseph W Sowka OD, Andrew S Gurwood OD and Alan Kabat OD, Jobson Publishing, with permission.

Table 2.1
Distinguishing features between the different types of conjunctivitis

	Most likely cause		Likely cause
	Bacterial (Fig. 2.1)	Allergic (Fig. 2.2)	Viral (Fig. 2.3)
Eyes affected	Both, but one eye affected a day or so before the other	Both	Both
Discharge	Purulent	Watery	Watery
Pain	Gritty feeling	Itching	Gritty feeling
Distribution of redness	Generalised and diffuse	Generalised but greatest in fornices	Generalised
Associated symptoms	None commonly	Rhinitis (might also have family history of atopy)	Cough and cold symptoms

Table 2.2
Specific questions to ask the patient: red eye

Question	Relevance
Other symptoms	• Symptoms of an upper respiratory tract infection suggest viral conjunctivitis • Vomiting suggests glaucoma
Visual changes	• Any loss of vision or haloes around objects should be viewed with extreme caution and suggests glaucoma or uveitis: **refer**
Pain/discomfort/itch	• True pain is associated with scleritis, keratitis, uveitis and acute glaucoma: **refer** • Pain described as a gritty/foreign body-type pain suggests conjunctivitis
Location of redness	• Redness concentrated near or around the coloured part of the eye suggests uveitis: **refer** • Generalised redness and redness towards the fornices (corner of the eyes) suggests conjunctivitis • Localised scleral redness suggests scleritis or episcleritis • Redness throughout the sclera suggests subarachnoid haemorrhage
Duration	• Any ocular redness (apart from subconjunctival haemorrhage and allergic conjunctivitis) lasting > 1 week requires referral

Unlikely causes

Episcleritis The eye appears red, although the colour is segmental and affects only part of the eye (Fig. 2.5). It is usually painless or a dull ache is felt. The condition is self-limiting, resolving in 6–8 weeks. It occurs most commonly in young women.

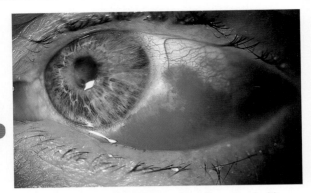

Figure 2.4 Subconjunctival haemorrhage. Reproduced with permission from *Clinical Ophthalmology*, 2003, by J Kanski, Butterworth-Heinemann, with permission.

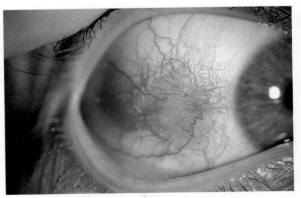

Figure 2.5 Episcleritis. Reproduced with permission from *Clinical Ophthalmology*, 2003, by J Kanski, Butterworth-Heinemann, with permission.

Scleritis Scleritis presents with similar symptoms as episcleritis but the condition is much more painful. It is often associated with autoimmune diseases, e.g. rheumatoid arthritis.

Keratitis (corneal ulcer) Corneal abrasion often results from trauma, administration of long-term steroid drops or overwear of soft contact lenses. Redness of the eye tends to be worse around the iris and pain can be very severe. The patient usually complains of photophobia accompanied by a watery discharge.

Uveitis Usually, only one eye is affected and the redness is localised to the limbal area (known as the ciliary flush). Photophobia and moderate to severe pain are usual. On examination, the pupil might appear irregularly shaped and constricted (Fig. 2.6). The patient might also complain of impaired reading. The likely cause is an antigen–antibody reaction and might occur as part of a systemic disease, such as rheumatoid arthritis or ulcerative colitis.

Very unlikely causes

Acute closed–angle glaucoma Eye pain is severe and the eye appears red and may be cloudy. Vision is blurred and the patient may notice haloes around lights. Onset can be very quick and characteristically occurs in the evening. Vomiting is often experienced due to the rapid rise in intra-ocular pressure.

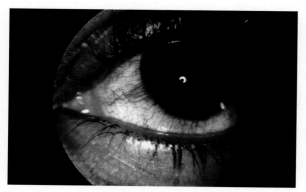

Figure 2.6 Uveitis. Reproduced from *Handbook of Ocular Disease Management* by Joseph W Sowka OD, Andrew S Gurwood OD and Alan Kabat OD, Jobson Publishing, with permission.

Primer for differential diagnosis of red eye

Figure 2.7 helps to differentiate between serious and non-serious ocular pathology.

Figure 2.7   Primer for differential diagnosis of red eye.

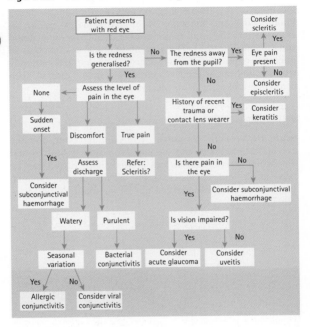

> ## TRIGGER POINTS indicative of referral: red eye
>
> - Associated vomiting.
> - Clouding of the cornea.
> - Distortion of vision.
> - Irregular-shaped pupil.
> - Photophobia.
> - Redness caused by a foreign body.
> - Redness localised around the pupil.
> - True eye pain.

Evidence of OTC medicine efficacy

Bacterial conjunctivitis (dibromopropamidine isethionate and propamidine)

Clinical trials are lacking to substantiate the effectiveness of these drugs in treating bacterial conjunctivitis. A further possible limitation of these products is the licensed dosage regimen of four times a day for drops, which has been reported to be too infrequent to achieve sufficient concentrations to kill or stop the growth of the infecting pathogen.

31

Allergic conjunctivitis

Avoiding the allergen will, in theory, result in control of symptoms. However, total avoidance is almost impossible and medication is usually necessary.

HINTS AND TIPS

Administration of eye drops: instructions to the patient
1. Wash your hands.
2. Tilt your head backwards, until you can see the ceiling.
3. Pull down the lower eyelid by pinching outwards to form a small pocket, and look upwards.
4. Holding the dropper in the other hand, hold it as near as possible to the eyelid without touching it.
5. Place one drop inside the lower eyelid then close your eye.
6. Wipe away any excess drops from the eyelid and lashes with the clean tissue.

Repeat steps 2 to 6 if more than one drop needs to be administered.

Administration of eye ointment: instructions to the patient
1. Repeat eye drop steps 1 and 2.
2. Pull down the lower eyelid.
3. Place a thin line of ointment along the inside of the lower eyelid.
4. Close your eye, and move the eyeball from side to side.
5. Wipe away any excess ointment from the eyelids and lashes using the clean tissue.

Your vision might be blurred after using ointment, but it will soon be cleared by blinking.

Mast cell stabilisers (e.g. sodium cromoglicate) have proven efficacy and are significantly better than placebo. In addition, the antihistamine levocabastine has shown to be significantly better than placebo and at least as effective as sodium cromoglicate. Sympathomimetics (e.g. naphazoline) do decrease ocular redness but can cause rebound redness with prolonged use, so, if used, they should be restricted to short-term use. A combination antihistamine/decongestant product is also available (Otrivine Antistin) but there are few trial data to support its effectiveness.

Based on evidence, both sodium cromoglicate and levocabastine are effective. Thus choice of product will depend on compliance. Levocabastine might be an appropriate first-line choice because it only requires twice-daily dosing, compared with four times a day for sodium cromoglicate.

Practical prescribing

Prescribing information relating to medication for red eye is summarised in the appendix.

Eyelid disorders

A number of disorders can afflict the eyelids, ranging from mild dermatitis to malignant tumours.

Arriving at a differential diagnosis

The most likely eyelid disorders seen in primary care will be blepharitis and styes. Practitioners should therefore direct questions to confirm one of these as the diagnosis as other eyelid problems are seen and listed below.

Probability	Cause
Most likely	Blepharitis, styes
Likely	Chalazion, contact irritant dermatitis
Unlikely	Entropion, ectropion
Very unlikely	Orbital cellulitis, carcinoma

Clinical features of blepharitis

Typically, blepharitis is bilateral with symptoms ranging from irritation and itching to burning, excessive tearing or skin flakes around the eyelashes (Fig. 2.8). Accompanying ocular symptoms include redness on the eyelid margins or missing or inturned lashes; the latter can lead to conjunctivitis.

Clinical features of styes

Patients will present with a swollen upper or lower lid, which will be painful and sensitive to touch. There might be associated conjunctivitis (Fig. 2.9). Styes are usually self-limiting and often spontaneously resolve.

The diagnosis of blepharitis or stye should be relatively straightforward providing a history is taken and an eye examination performed. Table 2.3 lists some of the questions to ask the patient to help confirm the diagnosis.

Conditions to eliminate

Likely causes

Chalazion   A chalazion has a similar appearance to a stye but will be painless. The lump should be clearly visible if the eyelid is everted. A chalazion is self-limiting but it may take a few weeks to resolve completely.

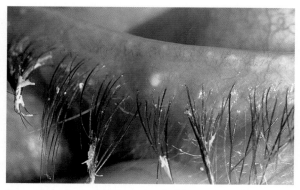

Figure 2.8   Blepharitis. Reproduced with permission from *Clinical Ophthalmology*, 2003, by J Kanski, Butterworth-Heinemann, with permission.

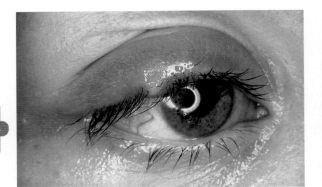

Figure 2.9 External stye. Reproduced with permission from *Clinical Ophthalmology*, 2003, by J Kanski, Butterworth-Heinemann, with permission.

Table 2.3
Specific questions to ask the patient: eyelid disorders

Question	Relevance
Age	<ul><li>Entropion and ectropion are associated with advancing age</li><li>Blepharitis, styes and dermatitis can affect all ages</li></ul>
Duration	<ul><li>A long-standing history of sore eyes suggests blepharitis, although it can be intermittent with periods of remission</li></ul>
Lid involvement	<ul><li>If the majority of the lid margin is inflamed and red then this suggests blepharitis</li><li>Localised lid involvement suggests a stye</li></ul>
Eye involvement	<ul><li>Ocular redness suggests blepharitis, entropion</li></ul>
Other coexisting conditions	<ul><li>Patients with blepharitis often have a history of other skin conditions, such as psoriasis or dandruff</li></ul>

Contact irritant dermatitis Many products, especially cosmetics, can be sensitising, leading to itching and flaking skin that mimics blepharitis. The patient should be questioned about recent use of such products to allow dermatitis to be eliminated.

Unlikely causes

Entropion Entropion refers to the in turning of the eyelid causing the eyelashes to be pushed against the cornea resulting in ocular irritation and conjunctival redness (Fig. 2.10). Referral is needed.

Ectropion Ectropion is the converse to entropion; the eyelid turns outwards, exposing the conjunctiva and cornea (Fig. 2.11). Patients will often complain of a continuously watering eye, but paradoxically this leads to dryness of the eye, as the eye is not receiving adequate lubrication.

Very unlikely causes

Orbital cellulitis Usually, orbital cellulitis is a complication from a sinus infection. The patient will be unwell and have

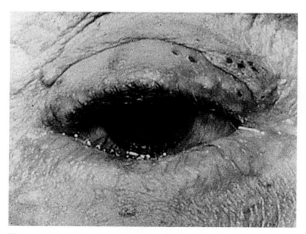

Figure 2.10 Entropion. Reproduced from *Handbook of Ocular Disease Management* by Joseph W Sowka OD, Andrew S Gurwood OD and Alan Kabat OD, Jobson Publishing, with permission.

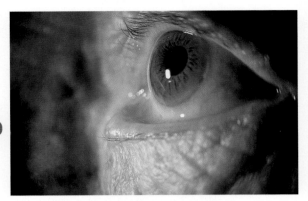

Figure 2.11 Ectropion. Reproduced from *Clinical Ophthalmology*, 2003, by J Kanski, Butterworth-Heinemann, with permission.

unilateral swollen eyelids. Eye movements might be restricted. Immediate referral is needed.

Basal cell carcinoma The lesion is usually nodular with a reddish hue (due to permanent capillary dilation) and most frequently affects the lower lid margin. No pain or discomfort is present and the patient will generally have a history of prolonged exposure to the sun.

> **❗ TRIGGER POINTS indicative of referral: blepharitis and styes**
>
> - Chalazion that becomes bothersome to the patient.
> - Inward- or outward-turning lower eyelid.
> - Middle-aged/elderly patient with painless nodular lesion on or near eyelid.
> - Patient with swollen eyelids and associated feelings of being unwell.

Evidence of OTC medicine efficacy

OTC medication is generally not required for blepharitis or styes. No specific products are available and both can respond well to conservative treatment, such as warm compresses.

Dry eye

A reduction in tear volume or alteration in tear composition causes dry eyes. It is a condition of the elderly and appears to affect women more than men.

Arriving at a differential diagnosis

The most likely cause of dry eyes in primary care is keratoconjunctivitis sicca (KCS) and is related to normal ageing. Other causes of dry eyes are possible and listed below.

Probability	Cause
Most likely	Related to the normal ageing process
Likely	Sjögren's syndrome, adverse drug reactions
Unlikely	Ectropion
Very unlikely	Bell's palsy

Clinical features of dry eye

Symptoms frequently reported are eyes that burn, feel tired, itchy, and irritated or gritty, although the eye will not be particularly red.

Table 2.4 lists some of the questions that should be asked to help determine the diagnosis.

Conditions to eliminate

Likely causes

Sjögren's syndrome   This syndrome is of unknown aetiology but is associated with rheumatic conditions. The patient experiences periods of exacerbation and remission – like KCS – but does not generally have a history of chronic dry eyes. It is also associated with dryness of other mucous membranes such as the mouth.

Table 2.4
Specific questions to ask the patient: dry eye

Question	Relevance
Duration	● A long-standing history of ocular irritation suggests KCS
Associated symptoms	● If no other symptoms are present then this suggests KCS ● Associated dry mouth suggests medication or an autoimmune disease
Amount of tears produced	● Watery eyes in a patient who complains that the eyes are dry suggest ectropion

Medicine-induced dry eye A number of medicines can exacerbate or produce side-effects of dry eyes; these are listed below:

● diuretics
● drugs that have an anticholinergic effect, e.g. tricyclic antidepressants (TCAs), antihistamines
● isotretinoin
● hormone replacement therapy.

Unlikely causes

Ectropion Sometimes the lower eyelid turns outwards. This overexposes the conjunctiva to the atmosphere leading to eye dryness (see Fig. 2.11).

Very unlikely causes

Bell's palsy Bell's palsy is characterised by unilateral facial paralysis, often with sudden onset. A complication of Bell's palsy is that the patient might be unable to close one eye or to blink, resulting in a decreased tear film and dry eye.

 TRIGGER POINTS indicative of referral: dry eye

● Associated dryness of mouth and other mucous membranes.
● Outward-turning lower eyelid.

Evidence of OTC medicine efficacy

Most medicines used to treat dry eye have no trial data to substantiate their effectiveness. Despite this, products such as hypromellose (e.g. Isopto Alkaline 1% and Isopto Plain 0.5%), polyvinyl alcohol (Hyoptears, Liquifilm Tears and Sno Tears) and wool fats (e.g. Lacri-Lube and Lubri-Tears) have been used for many years to good effect. Only carbomer 940 (e.g. Viscotears and GelTears) has trial data to show effectiveness for dry eye, being significantly better than placebo. In addition, a comparison trial between the two named examples showed them to be equally effective.

Practical prescribing

Prescribing information relating to medication for dry eye is summarised in the appendix.

HINTS AND TIPS

- Allergic reaction to preservatives: preservative-free hypromellose can be obtained if needed and single-unit dose vials (Artelac) are available.

Chapter 3

Otic conditions

Most ear conditions seen in primary care affect the middle and outer ear. External ear problems can usually be diagnosed via questioning and conducting a basic ear examination. Suspected middle ear problems should ideally be examined using an otoscope.

History taking

Without an otoscopical examination the practitioner is limited to the information that can be gained from questioning and a basic ear examination. However, certain symptoms can help decide what structure of the ear the problem originates from (Table 3.1).

Physical examination

After taking a history of the presenting complaint, the outer ear structures should be examined (Fig. 3.1). Initially, inspect the external ear for redness, swelling and discharge. Second,

Table 3.1
Ear symptoms and the affected ear structures

Symptom	External ear	Middle ear	Inner ear
Itch	✓		
Pain	✓	✓	
Discharge	✓	✓	
Deafness	✓	✓	✓
Dizziness			✓
Tinnitus			✓

Source: Acomb C, *Pharmaceutical Journal*, Aug 1991. Adapted with permission.

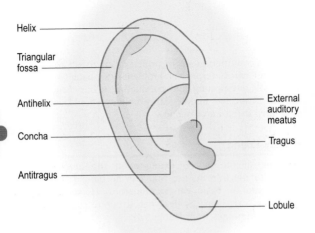

Figure 3.1 The pinna

apply pressure to the mastoid area (directly behind the pinna). Also move the pinna up and down and manipulate the tragus. This should provide some clues as the origin of the problem (Table 3.2).

Once the outer ear has been inspected, the ear canal should, if possible, be examined. In the absence of an oto-scope a pen torch could be used. Owing to the shape of the ear canal (the outer cartilaginous portion is upward and backward where as the inner bony portion is forward and downward) the pinna needs to be manipulated to obtain the best view of the ear canal (Fig. 3.2).

Ear wax impaction

Ear wax is the most common ear problem affecting the general population. Ears are self-cleaning and as such do not

Table 3.2
**Examination of the outer ear structures:
possible causes of presenting complaint**

Symptoms	Possible causes
Redness and swelling	● Perichondritis, haematoma
Discharge	● Otitis externa or otitis media ● Mucinous discharge originates from the middle ear (the ear canal has no mucous glands)
Pain in mastoid area	● Otitis media, mastoiditis
Pain when pressing tragus or moving pinna	● Otitis externa

need cleaning, although elderly people are more prone to ear wax owing to a decrease in cerumen-producing glands.

Arriving at a differential diagnosis

The most likely cause of ear wax impaction is misguided attempts by people to clean their ears. Practitioners should therefore direct questions to confirm this and to allow complications of ear wax impaction to be ruled out; these are listed below.

Probability	Cause
Most likely	Ear wax
Likely	Trauma of ear canal, foreign bodies (children)

Careful questioning accompanied by an inspection of the ear canal should allow the severity of ear wax impaction to be assessed and distinguish other conditions. Table 3.3 lists some of the questions that should be asked to aid diagnosis.

Clinical features of ear wax impaction

Patients usually have a history of gradual hearing loss and have varying degrees of ear discomfort and a feeling of fullness in the ear.

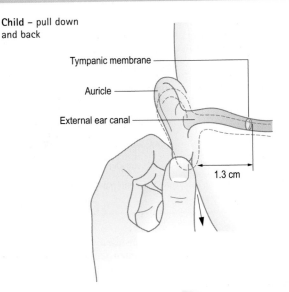

Child – pull down
and back

Tympanic membrane

Auricle

External ear canal

1.3 cm

44

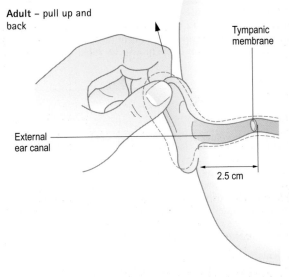

Adult – pull up and
back

Tympanic
membrane

External
ear canal

2.5 cm

Figure 3.2 Inspection of the ear canal in children and adults.

Table 3.3
Specific questions to ask the patient: ear wax

Question	Relevance
Associated symptoms	● Dizziness and tinnitus indicate an inner ear problem and should be referred ● Ear wax impaction rarely causes tinnitus, vertigo or true pain
History of trauma	● Check if the person has recently tried to clean the ears as this often leads to wax impaction
Use of medicines	● If a patient has used an appropriate OTC medication correctly this would necessitate referral for further investigation

Conditions to eliminate

Likely causes

Trauma of the ear canal It is common practice for people to use all manner of implements to try and clean the ear canal of wax (e.g. cotton buds, hairgrips, pens). Inspection of the ear canal might reveal laceration and the patient might experience greater conductive deafness due to the wax becoming further impacted.

Foreign bodies Symptoms can mimic ear wax impaction but, over time, discharge and pain is observed. Children are the most likely age group to present with a foreign body in the ear canal. Suspected cases need to be referred to a GP.

TRIGGER POINTS indicative of referral: ear wax

- Associated trauma related conductive deafness.
- Dizziness or tinnitus.
- Foreign body in the ear canal.
- OTC medication failure.
- Pain originating from the middle ear.

Evidence of OTC medicine efficacy

Cerumunolytics provide the mainstay of OTC treatment. Olive and almond oil along with sodium bicarbonate is still advocated by the *British National Formulary* (*BNF*) as being safe and efficacious, but this statement appears to be based more on anecdotal evidence than on published trial data. One double-blind study comparing Cerumol, sodium bicarbonate and water showed all three treatments to be significantly better than no treatment at all but there were no differences in efficacy between the treatment groups. Exterol has also been investigated (marketed as Otex to the general public) in a multicentre trial. The findings showed Exterol to be significantly better than its own vehicle and Cerumol. However, the study suffered from poor trial design, so the findings must be viewed with caution. Docusate sodium (Waxsol) has also been claimed to be highly efficacious, although these claims are unsubstantiated.

Practical prescribing

Prescribing information relating to medication for ear wax is summarised in the appendix.

HINTS AND TIPS

Administration of eardrops: instructions to the patient

1. Warm the solution in your hand for a few minutes prior to use as this makes insertion more comfortable.
2. Tilt your head to one side with the ear pointing towards the ceiling.
3. With one hand, straighten the ear canal (see Fig. 3.2).
4. Hold the dropper in the other hand and place the correct number of drops in to the ear canal without touching it.
5. Keep the head in the tilted position for several minutes (easiest to be lying down) or insert a cotton wool plug.
6. Once the head is returned to the normal position, wipe away any excess solution with a clean tissue.

Otitis externa

Otitis externa refers to generalised inflammation of the ear canal. It usually occurs as an acute episode and is common in patients following prolonged exposure of the ear to water (e.g. swimmer's ear).

Arriving at a differential diagnosis

The most likely cause of otitis externa in primary care is trauma related. Practitioners should therefore direct questions to confirm this as other causes of outer ear problems are seen and listed below.

Probability	Cause
Most likely	Trauma
Likely	Otalgia (from otitis media)
Unlikely	Perichondritis, haematoma
Very unlikely	Mastoiditis, malignant tumours

Clinical features of otitis externa

Otitis externa (Fig. 3.3) is characterised by irritation, which, depending on the severity, can become intense. This provokes the patient to scratch the skin of the ear canal, leading to trauma and pain. Manipulation of the tragus and pinna can exacerbate pain, as can chewing. Otorrhoea (ear discharge) follows and the skin of the ear canal can become oedematous, leading to conductive hearing loss.

Conditions to eliminate

Likely causes

Otalgia (earache)   Earache is normally due to a rapidly accumulating effusion in the middle ear (acute otitis media) and is most common in children aged 3–6 years. Throbbing ear pain and signs of infection are often present; the child may also appear unwell. Pain resolves on rupture of the tympanic membrane, which releases a mucopurulent discharge. An otoscopical (or pen torch) examination should show a red and bulging tympanic membrane. Children can develop recurrent otitis media, known as 'glue ear'.

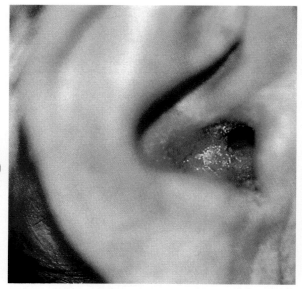

Figure 3.3 Otitis externa. Reproduced from *Shared Care for ENT*, 1999, by C Milford and A Rowlands, Isis Medical Media Ltd, with permission from Martin Dunitz Publishers.

Unlikely causes

Perichondritis In severe cases of otitis externa the inflammation can spread from the outer ear canal to the pinna, resulting in perichondritis (Fig. 3.4). Referral is needed.

Trauma Recent trauma (e.g. a blow to the head) can cause an auricular haematoma. This is often known as a cauliflower ear and requires non-urgent referral.

Very unlikely causes

Malignant tumours Basal and squamous cell carcinomas can develop on the pinna of the ear. Typically, these are slow growing and associated with increasing age. Any elderly patient with an ulcerative/crusting lesion must be referred.

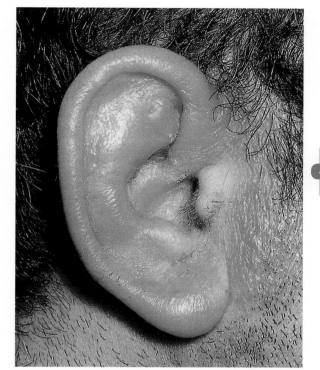

Figure 3.4 Perichondritis. From *Essential ENT Practice*, 1998, by R Corbridge, reproduced by permission of Hodder Arnold.

TRIGGER POINTS indicative of referral: otitis externa

- Ear pain in children under 6 years of age (within 24 hours).
- Generalised inflammation of the pinna.
- Symptoms persisting for 7 days or longer after initiation of treatment.
- Impaired hearing in children.
- Mucopurulent discharge.
- Pain on palpation of the mastoid area.
- Slow-growing growths on the pinna in elderly people.

Evidence of OTC medicine efficacy

OTC treatment of otitis externa is limited to oral antihistamines, to try and combat itching and irritation, or analgesia to control pain. The local analgesic effect of choline salicylate (available OTC as Earex Plus or Audax) has been compared with aspirin and paracetamol in two trials and was shown to reduce pain more quickly than oral analgesia.

An article in the *American Family Physician* (Sander et al 2001; 63: 927–936) stated that acidification of the ear canal using acetic acid combined with hydrocortisone was effective, but it is unclear whether the efficacy of the product is attributable to acetic acid, hydrocortisone or a combination of both. One OTC product, Earcalm Spray, contains 2% acetic acid and is indicated for the treatment of superficial infections of the ear canal. The *BNF* states that it might be useful to treat mild otitis externa, although there is a lack of trial data to support its use.

Practical prescribing

Prescribing information relating to medication for otitis externa is summarised in the appendix.

Chapter 4

Central nervous system (CNS)

The vast majority of patients will present with benign and non-serious conditions. Symptoms such as headache and insomnia are often brought on or worsened by pressure and stress. It is especially important then that social and work-related histories are taken when dealing with such requests.

Headache

Headache is a symptom of many different conditions. It can be the major presenting complaint (e.g. migraine) or one of many symptoms (e.g. upper respiratory tract infection).

Arriving at a differential diagnosis

When the presenting complaint is headache, the most likely cause in primary care for all age groups is tension headache. Practitioners should therefore direct questions to confirm this diagnosis as other causes of headache are seen and listed below.

Probability	Cause
Most likely	Tension headache
Likely	Migraine, sinusitis, eye strain
Unlikely	Cluster headache, temporal arteritis, trigeminal neuralgia, depression
Very unlikely	Glaucoma, meningitis, subarachnoid haemorrhage, raised intracranial pressure

Clinical features of tension headache

Pain is mild to moderate and described as non-throbbing, generalised and vice-like, or as a weight pressing down on the head. It usually affects the bifrontal or biooccipital regions and tends to worsen progressively through the day. Pressure or stress is known to worsen symptoms.

Despite the overwhelming majority of headaches in primary care being tension headaches, it is important to ensure that conditions needing doctor intervention are identified and referred. Table 4.1 lists some of the questions that should be asked to enable a correct diagnosis to be made.

Table 4.1
Specific questions to ask the patient: headache

Question	Relevance
Age/onset	● The likelihood of more serious causes of headache increases in patients > 50 years of age, especially if the patient has not experienced similar headache symptoms before. Mass lesions (tumours and haematoma) and temporal arteritis should be considered
	● Headache and fever at same time suggests infection
	● If the headache follows head trauma this suggests post-concussive headache or intracranial pathology: **refer**
Associated symptoms	● Nausea and/or vomiting in the absence of migraine-like symptoms suggests sinister pathology, e.g. mass lesions and subarachnoid haemorrhage: **refer**
	● Pain that increases when coughing/sneezing suggests sinusitis
	● Unilateral discharge/watery eye suggests cluster headache: **refer**
	● General malaise suggests temporal arteritis
Frequency and timing	● If associated with the menstrual cycle or at certain times, e.g. weekends or holidays, this suggests migraine
	● Headaches that occur in clusters at same time of day/night suggests cluster headache: **refer**
	● Headaches that occur on most days with same pattern suggests tension headache

Question	Relevance
Location of pain	• Nearly always unilateral in frontal, ocular or temporal area suggests cluster headache
	• Unilateral headache suggests migraine
	• Bilateral in frontal or occipital areas and described as a tight band suggests tension headache
	• Very localised pain suggests an organic cause: **refer**
Severity of pain	• Mild to moderate dull and band-like pain suggests tension headache
	• Severe to intense ache or throbbing pain suggests haemorrhage or aneurysm: **refer**
	• Piercing, boring, searing eye pain suggests cluster headache: **refer**
	• Moderate to severe throbbing pain that often starts as dull ache suggests migraine
Triggers	• Pain that worsens on exertion, coughing and bending suggests sinusitis or tumour
	• Food (10% of sufferers), menstruation and relaxation after stress suggest migraine
	• Pain worsening when lying down suggests cluster headache
Attack duration	• Typically, migraine attacks last between a few hours and 3 days
	• Tension headaches last between a few hours and several days (e.g. a week or more)
	• Pain lasting 2–3 hours suggests cluster headache

53

Conditions to eliminate

Likely causes

Migraine Pain tends to be unilateral, throbbing and moderate to severe. Almost all patients experience nausea but only a third will vomit. Patients often complain of photophobia, phonophobia and physical activity/movement intensifies the pain. Attacks last anything between a few hours and up to 3 days, with the average attack lasting 24 hours. Less than 25% of patients experience an aura before the onset of pain. Auras are visual or neurological and commonly include blind spots, zigzag lines, flashing and flickering lights or pins and needles. Migraine is three times more common than in women than men.

Sinusitis   The pain tends to be relatively localised, usually orbital, unilateral and dull. Bending down, coughing or sneezing often exacerbates the pain. The patient should have a history of recent cold symptoms.

Eye strain   Prolonged close work, for example operating a VDU, can cause frontal aching headache. Patients, in the first instance, should be referred to an optician for a routine eye check.

Unlikely causes

Cluster headache   Pain of cluster headache is described as intense, unilateral orbital boring pain. Typically, the headache occurs at the same time each day and lasts between 10 minutes and 3 hours. In approximately 50% of patients it wakes them 2–3 hours after falling asleep. Additionally, conjunctivitis and nasal congestion are experienced on the same side of the head as the headache. The condition is characterised by periods of acute attacks followed by periods of remission. It is six to nine times more common in men than in women. Refer to a doctor.

Temporal arteritis   Patients experience unilateral pain in the region of the temporal arteries (these run vertically up the side of the head, just in front of the ear). The arteries are tender to touch and might be visibly thickened. Fever, myalgia and general malaise are also usually present. It is most commonly seen in the elderly, especially women. Urgent referral is needed.

Trigeminal neuralgia   Pain follows the course of either the second or third division of the trigeminal nerve, and so is experienced in the cheek, jaws, lips or gums. The pain is short-lived, usually lasting only a couple of minutes, but is severe and lancing, and is almost always unilateral. Referral is needed.

Depression   Depression often presents with tension-like headaches. Check for loss of appetite, weight loss, decreased libido, sleep disturbances and constipation. If the patient exhibits these characteristics then referral to the GP would be necessary. Recent changes to the patient's social circumstances, for example loss of job, might also support your differential diagnosis.

Very unlikely causes

Acute closed–angle glaucoma   Headache is not usually the presenting symptom with glaucoma, although patients can suffer from a frontal headache as a result of severe eye pain. Vision is blurred and the cornea might look cloudy. In addition, patients might notice haloes around their vision. Vomiting is often experienced due to the rapid rise in intraocular pressure. Urgent referral is needed.

Meningitis   Severe generalised headache associated with fever, an obviously ill patient, neck stiffness and a purpuric rash are classically associated with meningitis. Early diagnosis of meningitis is notoriously difficult, and any child that has difficulty in placing the chin on the chest, has a headache and is running a temperature above 102°F (38.9°C) should be urgently referred.

Subarachnoid haemorrhage   The patient will experience very intense and severe pain, located in the occipital region. Nausea and vomiting are often present and a decreased lack of consciousness is prominent. Patients often describe the headache as the worse headache they have ever had. Urgent referral is needed.

Conditions causing raised intracranial pressure   Brain tumour, haematoma and abscess can give rise to varied headache symptoms, ranging from severe chronic pain to intermittent moderate pain. Pain can be localised or diffuse and tends to be more severe in the morning with a gradual improvement over the next few hours. Coughing, sneezing, bending and lying down can worsen the pain. Nausea and vomiting is common. Any patient with a recent history (last 2–3 months) of head trauma, headache of longstanding duration or insidious worsening of symptoms must be referred to a doctor.

Primer for differential diagnosis of headache

Figure 4.1 helps to aid differentiation of serious and non-serious causes of headache.

Figure 4.1 Primer for differential diagnosis of headache.

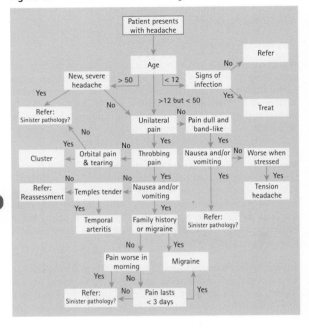

TRIGGER POINTS indicative of referral: headache

- Headache unresponsive to analgesics.
- Headache in children under 12 with stiff neck or skin rash.
- Headache occurs after recent (1–3 months) trauma injury.
- Headache that has lasted for more than 2 weeks.
- Nausea and/or vomiting in the absence of migraine symptoms.
- Neurological symptoms, if migraine excluded, especially change in consciousness.
- New or severe headache in patients over 50.
- Progressive worsening of headache symptoms over time.
- Symptoms indicative of cluster headache.
- Very sudden and/or severe onset of headache.

Evidence of OTC medicine efficacy

Analgesics (paracetamol, aspirin, ibuprofen)

All systemic analgesics, when prescribed as monotherapy, have proven efficacy in pain relief at standard doses.

Compound analgesics (paracetamol/codeine, aspirin/codeine or paracetamol/dihydrocodeine)

Codeine and dihydrocodeine can be prescribed OTC provided they are in combination with other analgesics. A number of papers have concluded that at OTC doses they are too low to produce statistically significant reductions in pain compared with single agents.

Products marketed specifically for the relief of migraine

Migraleve Pink tablets (paracetamol codeine combination [500/8] plus buclizine 6.25 mg)

A number of trials have investigated Migraleve Pink tablets against placebo, buclizine and ergotamine products. They have been shown to be superior to placebo in reducing the severity of attacks and as effective as Migril (which contains ergotamine) and buclizine.

Midrid (isometheptene mucate 65 mg and paracetamol 325 mg)

Trials conducted in the mid-1970s investigated isometheptene versus placebo and paracetamol. Midrid was superior to placebo and appeared to be better than paracetamol, but the benefit did not reach statistical significance. A further trial in 1978 (Behan, *Practitioner* 221: 937–939) compared Midrid against placebo and ergotamine. The trial concluded that Midrid was as effective as ergotamine and more beneficial than placebo, although it is unclear whether this was statistically significant.

From the trial data reviewed it appears that Midrid and Migraleve are more effective than placebo and similar to ergotamine preparations in reducing the severity of migraine attacks. Either could be recommended, but it is not known which product is most efficacious, as no comparison trials between the two products have been conducted.

Buccastem M (prochlorperazine 3 mg)
Trial data for prochlorperazine have shown it to be a potent antiemetic in a number of conditions, including migraine. It is administered via the buccal mucosa and therefore patients will need to be counselled on correct administration (see Hints and tips, below).

HINTS AND TIPS

Administration of buccal tablets: instructions to the patient
1. Place the tablet between either:
    a. the upper lip and gum above the front teeth or
    b. the cheek and upper gum.
2. Allow the tablet to dissolve slowly.
3. The tablet should take between 3 and 5 hours to dissolve.
4. If eating or drinking, place the tablet between the upper lip and gum, above the front teeth.
5. Touching the tablet with your tongue or drinking fluids may cause the tablet to dissolve faster.

Practical prescribing

Prescribing information relating to headache medication is summarised in the appendix.

Insomnia

Typically, an adult needs approximately 8 hours of sleep a day, although sleep requirements tend to decrease with age. Insomnia affects 20–40% of adults, with women being twice as likely to suffer as men. Insomnia is arbitrarily defined as transient (a few days), short-term (< 2–3 weeks) or chronic (> 3 weeks). Insomnia can have many causes (Table 4.2).

Arriving at a differential diagnosis

The most likely type of insomnia to be experienced is transient or short-term insomnia and usually results from changes in routine. Other causes of insomnia are seen in primary care and need to be eliminated before treatment is given.

58

Probability	Cause
Most likely	Changes to work hours, travel, noise disturbance
Likely	Insomnia in children, medicine-induced insomnia
Unlikely	Underlying medical conditions, depression

Table 4.2
The different causes of insomnia

Cause of insomnia	Example	Type of insomnia usually experienced
Altered work patterns	Shifts	Transient or short term
Poor sleep hygiene	Varying bed times	
The environment	Noise, foreign travel	
Psychological	Stress (exams, moving house)	Transient, short term or chronic depending on cause
Behavioural	Children (e.g. fear of the dark)	
Underlying medical conditions	Osteoarthritis	Chronic
Medication	Caffeine, decongestants	
Mental health	Depression	
Biological	Ageing, pregnancy	

Clinical features of insomnia

Patients will complain of difficulty in falling asleep or staying asleep, poor quality of sleep or of failure to feel refreshed after sleep.

The key to arriving at a differential diagnosis is to take a detailed sleep history. Two key features of insomnia need to

Table 4.3
Specific questions to ask the patient: insomnia

Question	Relevance
Pattern of sleep	● An emotional disturbance (predominantly anxiety) is associated with difficulty in falling asleep ● Falling asleep but awakening early and being unable to get back to sleep is sometimes associated with depression
Daily work routine	● Changes in work patterns, e.g. altered shift patterns and longer working hours, can precipitate insomnia
Underlying medical conditions	● Gastro-oesophageal reflux disease, pregnancy, pruritic skin conditions, asthma, Parkinson's disease, osteoarthritis and depression can all cause insomnia
Recent travel	● Time zone changes will affect a person's normal sleep pattern and it can take a number of days to re-establish normality

be determined: the type of insomnia and how it affects the person. Table 4.3 lists some of the questions that should be asked to help determine the cause of the insomnia.

Conditions to eliminate

Likely causes

Insomnia in children Bedwetting is the most common sleep arousal disorder in children. If this is not the cause then insomnia invariably stems from a behavioural problem, such as fear of the dark, insecurity or nightmares. Children should be referred to their GP for further evaluation.

Medicine-induced insomnia A number of medicines can cause insomnia:

● stimulants: caffeine (contained in chocolate, tea, coffee and cola drinks)

- theophylline, pseudoephedrine, monoamine oxidase inhibitors (MAOIs)
- antiepileptics (carbamazepine, phenytoin)
- alcohol (in excess or over long periods)
- propranolol (might cause nightmares)
- fluoxetine
- griseofulvin.

Unlikely causes

Underlying medical conditions It is necessary to take a medical history from the patient because many conditions can precipitate insomnia. A key role in these situations is to ensure that the patient's condition is being treated optimally and to check that the medication regimen is appropriate. If improvements to prescribing could be made then the prescriber should be contacted to discuss possible changes to the patient's medication.

Depression Between one- and two-thirds of patients suffering from chronic insomnia will have a recognisable psychiatric illness, most commonly depression. The patient will complain of having difficulty in staying asleep and suffer from early-morning waking. Other symptoms of depression, such as fatigue, loss of interest and appetite, feelings of guilt, low self-esteem, difficulty in concentrating and constipation, should be looked for.

Primer for differential diagnosis of insomnia

Figure 4.2 helps to aid diagnosis of insomnia.

 TRIGGER POINTS indicative of referral: insomnia

- Children under 12.
- Duration > 3 weeks.
- Insomnia for which no cause can be ascertained.
- Symptoms suggestive of anxiety or depression.

Evidence of OTC medicine efficacy

Transient and short-term insomnia should be initially managed by non-pharmacological measures. If these fail to

Figure 4.2   Primer for differential diagnosis of insomnia.

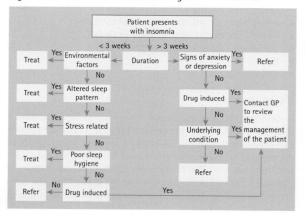

rectify the problem then short-term use of sedating antihistamines can be tried.

Sleep hygiene

The term 'sleep hygiene' is used to refer to patient behaviour and practice that affects sleep. Patients should be encouraged to maintain a routine, with a regular bedtime and wakening time. Food snacks and alcoholic and caffeine-containing drinks should also be avoided. Patients should avoid sleeping in very warm rooms and not exercise near bedtime. Elderly patients should also try to stop taking daytime naps as this further reduces the need to sleep at night.

Medication

The sedating antihistamines diphenhydramine and promethazine are the mainstay of OTC treatment.

Diphenhydramine (DPH)
A substantial body of evidence exists to support the clinical effectiveness of DPH as a sleep aid. DPH at doses of 50 mg has been shown to be consistently superior to placebo in inducing sleep, and as effective as 60 mg of sodium pentobarbital.

Promethazine

Promethazine is widely accepted to cause sedation when used for its licensed indications; however, only one trial appears to have been conducted investigating its use as a hypnotic (Adam et al, *Br J Clin Pharmacol* 1986; 22: 715–717). The conclusions from this small study (12 patients) stated that promethazine increased the length of sleep and sleep disturbances were reduced when compared with placebo.

Herbal remedies

Herbal remedies containing hops, German chamomile, skullcap, wild lettuce, passiflora and valerian are available and widely used. There is little evidence to support their use. The majority of information available in the literature relates to the hypothesised action of chemical constituents or studies in animals. Valerian appears to be the only product for which more than one trial has been conducted on humans, a number of which have reported a sedative effect.

Practical prescribing

Prescribing information relating to medication for insomnia is summarised in the appendix.

> **HINTS AND TIPS**
>
> ● Tolerance: tolerance might develop with continuous use of antihistamines. Treatment should therefore last no longer than 7–10 days.

Nausea and vomiting

Nausea and vomiting are common symptoms of many disorders, especially gastrointestinal conditions. Receptor cells in the walls of the gastrointestinal tract and parts of the nervous system reach a 'threshold value' that induces the vomiting reflex.

Arriving at a differential diagnosis

Most cases will have a gastrointestinal tract origin, with gastroenteritis being the most common acute cause in primary care in all age groups. Practitioners should therefore direct questions to confirm this diagnosis as other causes of nausea and vomiting are seen and listed below.

Probability	Cause
Most likely	Gastroenteritis (viral or bacterial)
Likely	Excess alcohol intake, pregnancy, migraine, medication, travel sickness (children)
Unlikely	Middle ear disorders
Very unlikely	Congenital abnormalities, pyloric stenosis, abdominal disorders (pancreatitis, renal colic, gastric ulcer)

64

Clinical features of gastroenteritis

Typical symptoms of gastroenteritis besides nausea/vomiting are diarrhoea, which might be bloody depending on the causative organism and abdominal discomfort. In children, viral gastroenteritis is common, but in this age group nausea/vomiting is associated with fever and otitis media.

Nausea and/or vomiting rarely occur in isolation. Other symptoms are usually present and should therefore allow a differential diagnosis to be made. Table 4.4 lists some of the questions that should be asked to help arrive at a differential diagnosis.

Conditions to eliminate

Likely causes

Excess alcohol consumption   The patient should always be asked about recent alcohol intake, as excess quantities are associated with nausea and early-morning vomiting.

Pregnancy   If nausea and vomiting occur in the absence of other symptoms in women of childbearing age pregnancy should always be considered. Sickness tends to be worse in the first trimester and in the early morning.

Migraine   Almost all patients experience nausea but only a third will vomit. Headache tends to be unilateral, throbbing and moderate to severe. Patients often complain of photo-

Table 4.4
Specific questions to ask the patient: nausea and vomiting

Question	Relevance
Onset	• If infective (bacterial causes), symptoms usually present within 48 hours of ingestion of contaminated food, although *Campylobacter* infection can take up to 96 hours to manifest • In migraine, alcohol and abdominal conditions onset of nausea/vomiting is usually quicker than with bacterial causes
Presence of abdominal pain	• Certain abdominal conditions, for example renal and biliary colic and pancreatitis, can cause nausea and vomiting • However, severe pain rather than nausea and/or vomiting will probably be the presenting symptom. The severity of the pain alone would trigger referral
Timing of nausea and vomiting	• Early-morning vomiting is often associated with pregnancy • Vomiting occurs immediately after food ingestion suggests gastritis • If vomiting begins 1 or more hours after eating food this suggests peptic ulcer

65

phobia and phonophobia, and physical activity/movement intensifies the pain.

Medicine-induced nausea and vomiting Many medications can cause nausea and vomiting. Cytotoxics, opiates, iron, antibiotics, non-steroidal anti-inflammatory drugs (NSAIDs), potassium supplements, selective serotonin reuptake inhibitors (SSRIs), nicotine gum (ingestion of nicotine rather than buccal absorption), theophylline and digoxin are associated with nausea.

Travel sickness Motion sickness is characterised by nausea, pallor and occasionally vomiting. Children between the ages of 2 and 12 are most commonly affected.

Unlikely causes

Middle ear diseases Any middle ear disturbance or imbalance can produce nausea and vomiting. If tinnitus, dizziness and vertigo are present this may suggest Ménière's disease, especially if only one ear is affected.

Very unlikely causes

Congenital abnormalities Vomiting in neonates (up to 1 month old) should always be referred as it suggests some form of congenital disorder, for example Hirschsprung's disease.

Pyloric stenosis If projectile vomiting occurs in infants under 3 months of age then pyloric stenosis should be considered.

Abdominal disorders (pancreatitis, renal colic, gastric ulcer) A number of gastrointestinal disorders present with nausea and/or vomiting. Patients who experience nausea/vomiting in association with abdominal pain are usually suffering from conditions that require GP intervention. Pain with such disorders is often severe and abrupt in onset.

TRIGGER POINTS indicative of referral: nausea and vomiting

- Severe abdominal pain.
- Suspected pregnancy.
- Unexplained nausea and vomiting in any age group.
- Vomiting in children under 1 year old.

Evidence of OTC medicine efficacy

Currently only domperidone (Motilium 10) and prochlorperazine (Buccastem M) have OTC licensed indications for the treatment of nausea and vomiting. In addition, sedating antihistamines and hyoscine are used for travel sickness.

Domperidone (Motilium 10)

Domperidone is licensed for the relief of postprandial symptoms that include nausea. A number of small studies suggest that domperidone is more effective than placebo. These studies were variable in design with differing inclusion criteria and methodology, making a definitive judgement on its effectiveness difficult to determine.

Prochlorperazine (Buccastem M)

Prochlorperazine is licensed for the relief of nausea and vomiting associated with migraine. It has proven efficacy in a number of conditions, including migraine, and represents a significant step forward in OTC treatment to manage migraine.

Medicines for travel sickness

First-generation sedating antihistamines (cyclizine, cinnarizine, meclozine and promethazine) and the anticholinergic hyoscine are routinely recommended to prevent motion sickness. All have shown various degrees of effectiveness, with hyoscine consistently proving the most effective.

Practical prescribing

Prescribing information relating to medication for nausea and vomiting is summarised in the appendix.

Chapter 5

Women's health

Women have unique healthcare needs ranging from pregnancy to menstrual disorders. A limited number of conditions can be managed appropriately with OTC medication.

Cystitis

Most patients self-diagnose cystitis, which is most common in the age group 15–34. It is thought that the patient's own bowel flora spread from the perineal and perianal areas is responsible for infection.

Arriving at a differential diagnosis

Acute uncomplicated cystitis will account for the majority of cases seen in primary care. Practitioners should therefore direct questions to confirm this diagnosis as other conditions can cause cystitis and are listed below.

Probability	Cause
Most likely	Acute uncomplicated cystitis
Likely	Pyelonephritis
Unlikely	Vaginitis, sexually transmitted diseases, oestrogen deficiency
Very unlikely	Medicine-induced cystitis

Clinical features of acute uncomplicated cystitis

Cystitis usually starts suddenly and is characterised by a combination of dysuria, urinary frequency (but only passing small amounts of urine), urgency, nocturia and haematuria. Low back pain and suprapubic discomfort might also be present but are uncommon.

To ensure other causes have been ruled out, Table 5.1 lists a number of questions that should be asked.

Table 5.1
Specific questions to ask the patient: cystitis

Question	Relevance
Duration	● Symptoms lasting > 5–7 days can develop into pyelonephritis: **refer**
Age of the patient	● Cystitis is unusual in children and might be a sign of a structural abnormality: **refer** ● Elderly female patients are more susceptible to complications associated with cystitis: **refer**
Presence of fever	● Fever associated with dysuria, frequency and urgency suggests an upper urinary tract infection: **refer**
Vaginal discharge	● The presence of vaginal discharge suggests vaginal infection
Location of pain	● Pain in the loin area suggests an upper urinary tract infection: **refer**

Conditions to eliminate

Likely causes

Pyelonephritis Involvement of higher anatomical urinary tract structures is the most frequent complication of cystitis. The patient will show signs of systemic infection such as fever, chills, flank pain and possibly nausea and vomiting. Referral is needed.

Unlikely causes

Vaginitis Vaginitis exhibits similar symptoms to cystitis, in that dysuria, nocturia and frequency are common, although vaginitis is associated with vaginal discharge. Irritants are frequently implicated in younger women, e.g. bubble baths. Symptoms are self-limiting and treatment unnecessary providing the irritant responsible is no longer used.

Sexually transmitted diseases (STDs) Symptoms are similar to cystitis but tend to be more gradual in onset and last longer. Pus in the urine is often seen and intermenstrual bleeding may be present.

Oestrogen deficiency   Postmenopausal women experience thinning of the endometrial lining due to a reduction in the levels of circulating oestrogen. This increases the likelihood of irritation or trauma leading to cystitis symptoms. Referral is appropriate if the symptoms recur.

Very unlikely causes

Medicine–induced cystitis   Non-steroidal anti-inflammatory agents (especially tiaprofenic acid) and cyclophosphamide have been shown to cause cystitis.

Primer for differential diagnosis of cystitis

Figure 5.1 helps to aid the differentiation of cystitis from other conditions.

TRIGGER POINTS indicative of referral: cystitis

- Children under 12.
- Elderly women.
- Duration longer than 7 days.
- Immunocompromised.
- Patients with associated fever, nausea, vomiting and flank pain.
- Pregnancy.
- Vaginal discharge.
- (Men).

Evidence of OTC medicine efficacy

Alkalinising agents (sodium citrate, sodium bicarbonate and potassium citrate)

There are few trial data to support the use of these agents; only one trial could be found to support their efficacy (Munday et al, *Genitourinary Med* 1990; 66: 461). This trial concluded that 80% of patients when treated with a 2-day course of Cymalon did gain symptomatic relief.

Figure 5.1 Primer for differential diagnosis of cystitis.

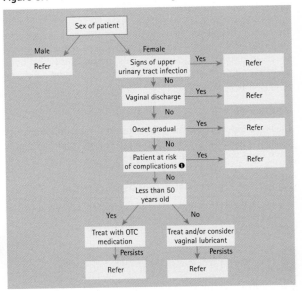

❶ At-risk patients: patients at risk of developing upper urinary tract infection include diabetics, pregnant women, the immunocompromised and the elderly.

Cranberry juice

A Cochrane review (Jepson et al, *Cochrane Database System Review* 2000; 2: CD001321) stated there was no reliable evidence to support the effectiveness of cranberry juice but Kontiokari et al (*BMJ* 2001; 32: 1571) found that cranberry concentrate did offer some protection against the recurrence of urinary tract infections, although not against acute attacks. Based on this latest trial it would appear that cranberry concentrate might offer some protection against urinary tract infections, but further trial data are needed before it should be recommended as a credible treatment.

Practical prescribing

Prescribing information relating to medication for cystitis is summarised in the appendix.

HINTS AND TIPS

- OTC treatment failure: all marketed products are presented as a 2-day treatment course; treatment failure warrants referral. Trimethoprim 200 mg twice daily would be a suitable treatment and has been used under patient group direction by nurses (for online information, see www.druginfozone.nhs.uk/pgd/ DisplayProtocol.asp?ID=721).

Vaginal discharge

Patients of any age can experience vaginal discharge, and it has been reported that 75% of all women will experience at least one episode of thrush during their childbearing years. Thrush is uncommon in prepubertal girls unless they have been receiving antibiotics. In adolescents it is the second most common cause of vaginal discharge after bacterial vaginosis.

Arriving at a differential diagnosis

The most likely cause of vaginal discharge in primary care is thrush. Practitioners should therefore direct questions to confirm this diagnosis as other conditions can cause vaginal discharge and are listed below.

Probability	Cause
Most likely	Thrush
Likely	Bacterial vaginosis, trichomoniasis, medicine-induced thrush
Unlikely	Atrophic vaginitis, cystitis, mixed infection, diabetes, pregnancy, irritants

Clinical features of thrush

The dominant feature of thrush is vaginal itching. This is often accompanied by soreness of the vulval lips and discharge in up to 20% of patients. The discharge has little or no odour and is curd-like. Symptoms are generally acute in onset. Table 5.2 highlights the similarities and differences of

Table 5.2
Presenting symptoms of the three commonest causes of vaginal discharge

	Discharge	*Odour*	*Itch*
Thrush	White curd or cottage-cheese-like	Little or none	Prominent
Bacterial vaginosis	White and thin	Strong and fishy	Slight
Trichomoniasis	Green–yellow and frothy	Malodorous	Slight

the three most commonly encountered conditions that cause vaginal discharge.

Conditions to eliminate

Likely causes

Bacterial vaginosis   The exact cause of bacterial vaginosis is unknown, although *Gardnerella vaginalis* is often implicated. Roughly 50% of patients will have a thin white discharge with a strong fishy odour, which might be worse during menses and after coitus.

Trichomoniasis   Trichomoniasis, a protozoan infection, is primarily transmitted through sexual intercourse. Women usually present with profuse, frothy, greenish-yellow and malodorous discharge accompanied by vulvar itching. Other symptoms include vaginal spotting, dysuria and urgency.

Medicine–induced thrush   Broad-spectrum antibiotics, corticosteroids and medication affecting the oestrogen status of the patient (oral contraceptives, hormone replacement therapy, tamoxifen and raloxifene) can predispose women to thrush.

Unlikely causes

Atrophic vaginitis   Symptoms consistent with thrush in elderly women, especially vaginal itching and burning, might be due to atrophic vaginitis. Refer to the GP.

Cystitis Dysuria might affect up to one in three women with vaginal infection. However, the patient will often be able to sense that it is an external discomfort, rather than an internal discomfort located in the urethra or bladder.

Mixed infection It has been reported that 14% of women have mixed infections of thrush, bacterial vaginosis or trichomoniasis. OTC treatment failure with an antifungal should warrant referral to exclude a mixed infection.

Diabetes Patients with poorly controlled or undiagnosed diabetes (type 1 or 2) are more likely to suffer from thrush because hyperglycaemia can enhance production of protein surface receptors on *Candida albicans* organisms. This hinders phagocytosis by neutrophils, thus making thrush more difficult to eliminate.

Pregnancy Hormonal changes during pregnancy will alter the vaginal environment and have been reported to make eradication of *Candida* more difficult.

Chemical and mechanical irritants Ingredients in feminine hygiene products, for example bubble baths, vaginal sprays and douches, might precipitate attacks of thrush by altering vaginal pH. Condoms have also been found to irritate and alter the vaginal pH.

75

Primer for differential diagnosis of vaginal thrush

Figure 5.2 helps to aid the differentiation of vaginal thrush.

> ❗ **TRIGGER POINTS indicative of referral: thrush**
>
> - Diabetics.
> - Discharge that has a strong smell.
> - OTC medication failure.
> - Pregnant women.
> - Recurrent attacks.
> - Women under 16 and over 60.

Figure 5.2 Primer for differential diagnosis of vaginal thrush.

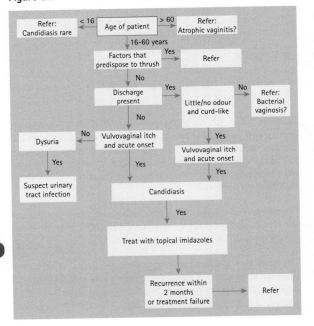

Evidence of OTC medicine efficacy

Topical therapy (imidazoles, e.g. clotrimazole, econazole, miconazole)

All the antifungals used to treat vaginal thrush have proven and comparable efficacy with clinical cure rates of approximately 80%. Additionally, cure rates between single or multiple dose therapy and multiple day therapy are also clinically equivalent. Treatment choice will therefore be driven by patient acceptability.

Systemic therapy (fluconazole)

Fluconazole has equal cure rates to topical imidazoles and a Cochrane review (Watson et al, Cochrane Library issue 2, 2004) recommended it as treatment of choice for non-pregnant women. Although more convenient than pessaries, the high cost and increased side-effect profile might dissuade people from buying these products.

Practical prescribing

Prescribing information relating to medication for vaginal thrush is summarised in the appendix.

HINTS AND TIPS

- Symptom resolution: the symptoms of thrush, such as burning, soreness or itching of the vagina, should disappear within 3 days of treatment. If no improvement is seen after 7 days the patient should see the GP.
- Vaginal douching: this should not be encouraged and avoided wherever possible.
- Yoghurt: some people recommend live yoghurt as a 'natural' treatment. The evidence of the usefulness of yoghurt is conflicting. However, as no harm would come to a patient who chose to use yoghurt then, providing suitable pharmacological measures are taken, there is currently no strong evidence to discourage its use.

77

Administration of pessaries: instructions to the patient

1. As the dosage is at night, you should use the pessary when in bed.
2. Remove the pessary from the packaging and place firmly into applicator (the end of the applicator needs to be gently squeezed to allow the pessary to fit).
3. Lying on your back, with your knees drawn towards the chest, insert the applicator as deeply as is comfortable into the vagina.
4. Slowly press the plunger of the applicator until it stops. Remove and dispose of the applicator.
5. Remain in the supine position.

Period pain

Menstruation spans the years between menarche to menopause. Typically, menstruation will start around the age of 12 and cease at approximately 50. Period pain affects

30–60% of menstruating women, with 1 in 10 reporting severe and debilitating pain. It is classically associated with young women who have recently started having regular periods. However, there might be a gap of months or years between menarche and onset of symptoms. This is important to know, as anovulatory cycles are usually pain free.

Arriving at a differential diagnosis

The most likely cause of period pain seen in primary care is primary dysmenorrhoea. Practitioners should therefore direct questions to confirm this as other conditions cause period pain and are listed below.

Probability	Cause
Most likely	Primary dysmenorrhoea
Likely	Secondary dysmenorrhoea (endometriosis)
Unlikely	Pelvic inflammatory disease, medication, dysfunctional uterine bleeding
Very unlikely	Endometrial carcinoma

Clinical features of primary dysmenorrhoea

A typical presentation of primary dysmenorrhoea is of lower abdominal cramping pains shortly before (6 hours) and for 2 or possibly 3 days after the onset of bleeding. Associated back pain, nausea and/or vomiting can also occur in up to 50% of patients.

To establish the diagnosis, the frequency, severity and relationship of symptoms to the menstrual cycle need to be established. Table 5.3 lists some of the questions that should be asked to help to determine if referral is needed.

Conditions to eliminate

Likely causes

Endometriosis (presence of endometrial tissue outside of the uterus) Endometriosis is the most common cause of secondary dysmenorrhoea. Patients experience lower abdominal aching pain that starts 5–7 days before menstruation. Pain

Table 5.3
**Specific questions to ask the patient:
primary dysmenorrhoea**

Question	Relevance
Age	• < 20 years suggests primary dysmenorrhoea • > 30 years suggests secondary dysmenorrhoea
Nature of pain	• Cramping pain suggests primary dysmenorrhoea • Pain described as dull, continuous diffuse pain suggests secondary causes
Severity of pain	• Pain that is mild/moderate suggests primary dysmenorrhoea • Severe lower abdominal pain suggests endometriosis or pelvic inflammatory disease
Onset of pain	• Pain that starts shortly before the onset of menses suggests primary dysmenorrhoea • Pain that starts a few days before the onset of menses suggests a secondary cause

79

often worsens at the onset of menstruation and can be constant and severe. Referred pain into the back and down the thighs is also possible.

Unlikely causes

Dysfunctional uterine bleeding   'Dysfunctional uterine bleeding' is a non-specific medical term defined as abnormal uterine bleeding that is not due to structural or systemic disease. The majority of cases are attributable to menorrhagia (heavy periods) and the patient will also suffer from cramping pain. Patients should be asked if their periods are different from usual.

Pelvic inflammatory disease   Pelvic inflammatory disease is associated with lower abdominal pain; however, other symptoms, such as fever, malaise, vaginal discharge and dyspareunia, are present.

Medicine-induced menstrual bleeding   A number of medicines are thought to cause uterine bleeding and associated pain. These are listed below:

- anticoagulants
- cimetidine
- monoamine oxidase inhibitors
- phenothiazines
- steroids
- thyroid hormones
- intrauterine devices.

Very unlikely causes

Endometrial carcinoma   This is characterised by inappropriate uterine bleeding and usually occurs in postmenopausal women. All unexplained bleeding in postmenopausal women should be referred, as up to a third of cases are due to endometrial carcinoma.

80

> ❗ **TRIGGER POINTS indicative of referral: primary dysmenorrhoea**
>
> - Heavy or unexplained bleeding.
> - Pain experienced before menses.
> - Pain that increases at the onset of menses.
> - Signs of systemic infection (e.g. fever, malaise).
> - Vaginal bleeding in postmenopausal women.
> - Women over the age of 30.

Evidence of OTC medicine efficacy

Non-steroidal anti-inflammatory drugs would be a logical choice because raised prostaglandin levels cause primary dysmenorrhoea. In multiple clinical trials these agents have been shown to be effective in 80–85% of women. Other products marketed for primary dysmenorrhoea include hyoscine butylbromide (Buscopan) and hyoscine hydrobromide (Feminax). Although both products are marketed for primary dysmenorrhoea, there appears to be little or no evidence to support the manufacturers' claims. Only one trial involving Buscopan was found and this study failed to demonstrate a significant effect compared with placebo, or its comparator drug aspirin (Kemp, *Curr Med Res Opin* 1972; 1: 19–25).

> **HINTS AND TIPS**
>
> - Effectiveness of treatment: a trial of two to three cycles should be long enough to determine if therapy with non-steroidal anti-inflammatory drugs is successful.

Practical prescribing

Prescribing information relating to medication for period pain is summarised in the appendix.

Premenstrual syndrome

'Premenstrual syndrome' is a broad term with varying definitions encompassing a wide range of symptoms – both physical and psychological. It appears mostly to affect women aged in their 30s and 40s.

Arriving at a differential diagnosis

Due to the varying and wide-ranging symptoms associated with premenstrual syndrome, a diagnosis can be difficult to establish. Other gynaecological and mental health disorders seen in primary care need to be ruled out.

Probability	Cause
Most likely	Premenstrual syndrome
Likely	Mental health problems
Unlikely	Primary dysmenorrhoea

Clinical features of premenstrual syndrome

The most common psychological symptoms of premenstrual syndrome are irritability, agitation, nervousness and anxiety. Physiological symptoms experienced are breast tenderness, bloating, water retention, abdominal pain and headache. Symptoms are experienced 7–14 days before menses (around the time of ovulation) and disappear shortly after bleeding starts. Gaining information over the previous three cycles rather than the presenting symptoms should allow a fuller picture of symptoms to be gained.

Conditions to eliminate

Likely causes

Mental health disorders   Depression and anxiety are common mental health disorders, which often go undiagnosed. Patients with premenstrual syndrome might experience similar symptoms, such as low or sad mood, loss of interest or pleasure and prominent anxiety or worry. Other symptoms might include disturbed sleep and appetite, dry mouth and poor concentration. However, symptoms are not cyclical and are not associated with some of the physiological symptoms of premenstrual syndrome, such as breast tenderness and bloatedness.

Unlikely causes

Primary dysmenorrhoea   The abdominal pain of primary dysmenorrhoea and that experienced by premenstrual syndrome sufferers can be similar. However, the symptoms of premenstrual syndrome tend to be present for longer in the cycle before the menses, and to subside more quickly after the menses than in primary dysmenorrhoea. Additionally, psychological symptoms may be present with premenstrual syndrome and the symptoms tend to occur in older women.

82

> ❗ TRIGGER POINTS indicative of referral: premenstrual syndrome
>
> - Psychological symptoms alone.
> - Severe or disabling symptoms.
> - Symptoms that either worsen or stay the same after the onset of menses.
> - Women under the age of 30.

Evidence of OTC medicine efficacy

A number of dietary supplements are marketed for premenstrual syndrome-like symptoms. Most notably, vitamin B_6 has been widely touted as an effective therapy. A recent review (*BMJ* 1999; 318: 1375–1381) concluded that symptoms of irritability, fatigue and bloating were favourably reduced with vitamin B_6 supplementation. Other dietary supplements, e.g. vitamin E, magnesium, evening primrose oil and calcium, have been advocated. Only calcium supplementation at doses of 1200–1600 mg per day appear to have any evidence of efficacy.

Practical prescribing

Prescribing information relating to medication for premenstrual syndrome is summarised in the appendix.

Chapter 6

Gastroenterology

The main function of the gastrointestinal tract is to break food down in to a suitable energy source to allow normal physiological function of cells. Needless to say, the process is complex and involves many different organs. Consequently, there are many conditions that affect the gastro-intestinal tract. Some of these are acute and self-limiting, and respond well to OTC medication; others are serious and require referral.

The oral cavity

The oral cavity comprises the cheeks, hard and soft palates and tongue. The tongue and cheeks position large pieces of food so teeth can tear and crush food into smaller particles. Saliva moistens, lubricates and begins to digest carbohydrates prior to swallowing.

The physical exam

The oral cavity (Fig. 6.1) can easily be examined provided the mouth can be viewed with a good light source, preferably a pen torch.

The basic steps for performing a simple examination of the mouth are as follows:

1. Wash your hands.
2. Examine the lesions/problem area of the oral cavity that the person has presented with.
3. Once checked, inspect the rest of the oral cavity. Look for:
   a. signs of bleeding gums
   b. other ulcerated/sore areas of the mouth.
4. The floor of the mouth and underside of the tongue can be viewed by asking the patient to curl the tongue towards the roof of the mouth.
5. The buccal mucosa is best observed when the patient half opens the mouth.

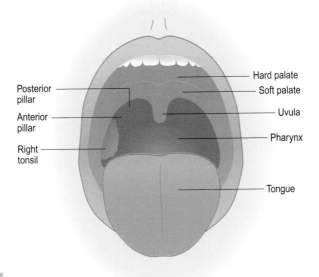

Hard palate

Soft palate

Posterior
pillar

Uvula

Anterior
pillar

Pharynx

Right
tonsil

Tongue

86

Figure 6.1 The oral cavity.

Mouth ulcers

Mouth ulcers are common. It is estimated that one in five of
the general population is affected, although no one theory
is accepted as to their cause. Stress, trauma, food hyper-
sensitivities, nutritional deficiencies (iron, zinc and vitamin
B_{12}) and infection have all been implicated.

Arriving at a differential diagnosis

The most likely cause of ulcers encountered in primary care
is minor aphthous ulcers. Practitioners should therefore
direct questions to confirm this diagnosis as other conditions
that cause ulcers are seen and listed below.

Probability	Cause
Most likely	Minor aphthous ulcers
Likely	Major aphthous ulcers, trauma
Unlikely	Herpetiform ulcers, herpes simplex, oral thrush
Very unlikely	Squamous cell carcinoma, erythema multiforme (Stevens–Johnson syndrome), Behçet's syndrome

Clinical features of minor aphthous ulcers

The ulcers of minor aphthous ulcers are shallow, roundish, grey–white in colour and painful. They are small, usually less than 1 cm in diameter, and occur singly or in small crops of up to five ulcers (Fig. 6.2). Ulcers heal in 7–14 days.

Although it is likely the patient will be suffering from minor ulcers, it is essential that other causes are recognised and appropriate referrals made to the GP. Table 6.1 lists some of questions that should be asked to aid diagnosis. After asking questions the oral cavity should be inspected to confirm the diagnosis.

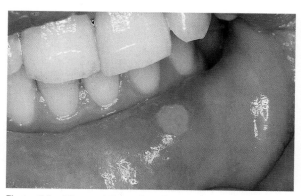

Figure 6.2 Minor aphthous ulcer. Reproduced from *Cawson's Essentials of Oral Pathology and Oral Medicine* by R Cawson et al, 2002, Churchill Livingstone, with permission.

Table 6.1
**Specific questions to ask the patient:
mouth ulcers**

Question	Relevance
Number of ulcers	<ul><li>Single or ulcers in small crops suggests minor ulcers</li><li>A single, large, ulcerated area suggests more serious pathology: **refer**</li><li>Numerous ulcers suggest herpetiform or herpes simplex ulcers</li></ul>
Location of ulcers	<ul><li>Ulcers on the side of the cheeks tongue and inside of the lips suggest minor ulcers</li><li>Ulcers located towards the back of the mouth suggest major or herpetiform ulcers</li></ul>
Size and shape	<ul><li>Irregular-shaped ulcers suggest trauma</li><li>Pinpoint ulcers suggest herpetiform ulcers</li><li>Large ulcers suggest major ulcers or oral thrush</li></ul>
Associated pain	<ul><li>A painless ulcer suggests sinister pathology: **refer**</li></ul>
Age (with no previous history)	<ul><li>Age < 10 years suggests primary infection with herpes simplex</li><li>Age 10–50 years suggests minor ulcers</li><li>Age > 50 years suggests sinister pathology</li></ul>

88

Conditions to eliminate

Likely causes

Major aphthous ulcers   Characterised by large (greater than 1 cm in diameter) ulcers, in crops of 10 or more. The ulcers often coalesce to form one large ulcer. The ulcers heal slowly and may persist for many weeks (Fig. 6.3).

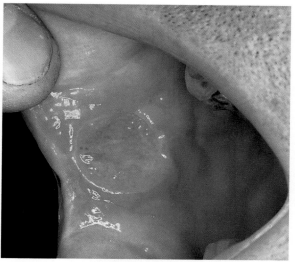

Figure 6.3 Major aphthous ulcer. Reproduced from *Cawson's Essentials of Oral Pathology and Oral Medicine* by R Cawson et al, 2002, Churchill Livingstone, with permission.

Trauma Trauma to the oral mucosa is most commonly associated with biting the tongue or inside of the mouth, resulting in ulcers with an irregular border (Fig. 6.4).

Unlikely causes

Herpetiform ulcers Ulcers are pinpoint and occur in large crops of up to 100 at a time often in the posterior part of the mouth. They usually heal within a month (Fig. 6.5).

Herpes simplex Herpes simplex virus is a common cause of oral ulceration in children. Ulcers can occur in any part of the oral mucosa, especially the gums, tongue and cheeks. The ulcers tend to be small and many in number. Prior to the eruption of ulcers, the person might show signs of systemic infection, such as fever and pharyngitis.

Oral thrush Oral thrush usually presents as creamy-white soft elevated patches. It can occur anywhere in the oral

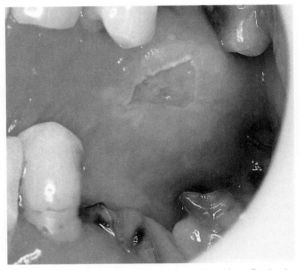

Figure 6.4 Ulcer caused by trauma. Reproduced from *Textbook of General and Oral Medicine* by D Wray et al, 1999, Churchill Livingstone.

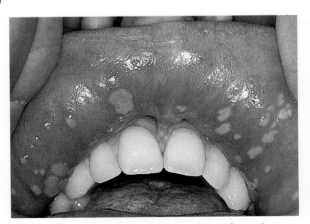

Figure 6.5 Herpetiform ulcer. Reproduced from *Cawson's Essentials of Oral Pathology and Oral Medicine* by R Cawson et al, 2002, Churchill Livingstone, with permission.

cavity and can be wiped off, revealing underlying erythematous mucosa. Pain and soreness are often present.

Very unlikely causes

Squamous cell carcinoma Approximately 2000 people in the UK are diagnosed with squamous cell carcinoma each year, and smokers account for 75% of cases. Initially the ulcer is painless, but over time it becomes painful. The majority are noted on the side of the tongue, mouth and lower lip. The ulcer is likely to have been present for a number of weeks before the patient seeks help.

Erythema multiforme Symptoms are sudden in onset, causing widespread ulceration of the oral cavity, with the lips commonly bloody and crusted. In addition, the patient may have a skin rash located towards the extremities (e.g. palms and soles). Conjunctivitis is common is Stevens–Johnson syndrome, a severe form of erythema multiforme.

Behçet's syndrome Patients who suffer from recurrent, painful major aphthous ulcers accompanied by lesions in the genital region and eye involvement (iridocyclitis) may have Behçet's syndrome.

91

Primer for differential diagnosis of mouth ulcers

Figure 6.6 helps to aid differentiation between serious and non-serious conditions associated with oral lesions.

TRIGGER POINTS indicative of referral: mouth ulcers

- Children under 10 years.
- Duration longer than 14 days.
- Painless ulcer.
- Signs of systemic illness, e.g. fever.
- Ulcers greater than 1 cm in diameter.
- Ulcers in crops of 5–10 or more.

Evidence of OTC medicine efficacy

There are numerous OTC treatments for the temporary relief and treatment of mouth ulcers, including corticosteroids, local anaesthetics, astringents and antiseptics.

Figure 6.6 Primer for differential diagnosis of mouth ulcers.

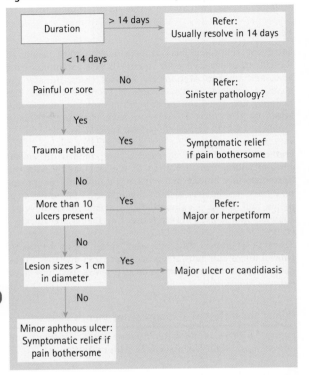

Corticosteroids (triamcinolone acetonide in Orabase and hydrocortisone sodium succinate pellets)

Corticosteroids have been suggested as useful preparations to treat minor ulcers by a number of authors, yet clinical evidence from trial data is not strong. Small trials involving both preparations appear to help relieve pain but do not speed up healing.

Products containing anaesthetic or analgesics

There are very few trial data to support the pain-relieving effect of anaesthetics or analgesics in minor ulcers, apart from choline salicylate. However, these preparations are clinically effective in other painful oral conditions. It is therefore not unreasonable to expect some relief of symptoms to be shown when these products are used.

Practical prescribing

Prescribing information relating to medication for ulcers is summarised in the appendix.

Oral thrush

The very young and the very old are most likely to suffer from oral thrush, and it has been reported that 5% of newborn infants and 10% of debilitated elderly patients suffer from oral thrush.

Arriving at a differential diagnosis

The most likely cause of white patches in the oral cavity seen in primary care is thrush. Practitioners should therefore direct questions to confirm this diagnosis as other conditions can cause oral lesions; these are listed below.

Probability	Cause
Most likely	Thrush
Likely	Minor aphthous ulcers, medicine induced, ill-fitting dentures
Unlikely	Underlying medical disorders, e.g. diabetes, xerostomia (dry mouth) and immunosuppression
Very unlikely	Leukoplakia, squamous cell carcinoma

Clinical features of oral thrush

Oral thrush can occur anywhere in the oral cavity and appears as soft, creamy-white, elevated patches that can be wiped off to reveal the underlying erythematous mucosa. Pain and soreness are often present.

Oral thrush is relatively straightforward to diagnose providing a number of questions are asked to eliminate underlying pathology and exclude risk factors (Table 6.2).

Table 6.2
Specific questions to ask the patient: oral thrush

Question	Relevance
Size and shape of lesion	● Irregular-shaped lesions suggest thrush, trauma ulcers or leukoplakia ● Pinpoint lesions suggest herpetiform ulcers ● Large lesions suggest major ulcers or oral thrush
Associated pain	● Painless lesions suggest a sinister pathology ● Painful lesions suggest thrush or ulcers
Location of lesions	● Lesions on the tongue and cheeks suggest thrush ● Lesions on the pharynx suggest drug-induced problems associated with inhaled corticosteroids

After questioning, the oral cavity should be inspected to confirm the diagnosis.

Conditions to eliminate

Likely causes

Minor aphthous ulcers   Minor aphthous ulcers are shallow, roundish, grey–white in colour and painful. They are small – usually less than 1 cm in diameter – and occur singly or in small crops of up to five ulcers. The ulcers heal in 7–14 days.

Medicine induced   Broad-spectrum antibiotics and inhaled corticosteroids can precipitate oral thrush by altering the normal flora of the oral cavity. If corticosteroids are the cause then patients should be encouraged to use a spacer and wash their mouth out after using the inhaler to minimise this problem.

Ill-fitting dentures   Poorly fitting dentures will cause local trauma to the surrounding epithelium, resulting in erythema and pain.

Unlikely causes

Underlying medical disorders   A number of conditions (e.g. diabetes) will predispose the patient to candidiasis either because the oral environment becomes more favourable to *Candida* or because the patient's immune defences are weakened, allowing opportunistic infection to occur.

Very unlikely causes

Leukoplakia   Leukoplakia is a precancerous state that presents as a symptomless white patch, typically in people over the age of 50. Unlike oral thrush, the patch cannot be wiped off. All elderly patients presenting with such symptoms should be referred.

Squamous cell carcinoma   Initially, the ulcer is painless but over time it becomes painful. The majority are noted on the side of the tongue, mouth and lower lip. The ulcer is likely to have been present for a number of weeks before the patient seeks help.

Primer for differential diagnosis of oral thrush

Figure 6.7 helps to differentiate thrush from other oral lesions.

TRIGGER POINTS indicative of referral: oral thrush

- Diabetics.
- Duration > 3 weeks.
- Immunocompromised patients.
- Painless lesions.

HINTS AND TIPS

- Application of Daktarin: patients should be advised to hold the gel in the mouth for as long as possible to increase contact time between the medicine and the infection.
- Duration of treatment: treatment should be continued for up to 2 days after the symptoms have cleared to prevent relapse and reinfection.

Figure 6.7 Primer for differential diagnosis of oral thrush.

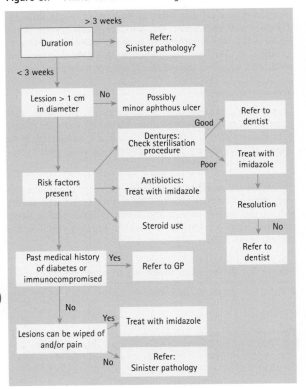

Evidence of OTC medicine efficacy

Only Daktarin oral gel (miconazole) is available OTC. It has proven efficacy and appears to have clinical cure rates of between 80% and 90%.

Practical prescribing

Prescribing information relating to miconazole is summarised in the appendix.

Gingivitis

Gingivitis simply means inflammation of the gums and is caused by an excess build-up of plaque on the teeth. The condition is prevented by regular tooth brushing.

Arriving at a differential diagnosis

The most likely cause of gingivitis seen in primary care is poor oral hygiene, which, if untreated, can result in long-term problems. Practitioners should therefore direct questions to confirm this diagnosis as other conditions can cause inflammation of the gums and are listed below.

Probability	Cause
Most likely	Gingivitis
Likely	Periodontitis
Unlikely	Medicine-induced gum bleeding
Very unlikely	Agranulocytosis and leukaemia

Clinical features of gingivitis

97

Gingivitis can go unnoticed because symptoms can be mild and painless but patients might notice that the gums are redder, swollen and bleed easily with slight trauma, e.g. when brushing teeth. Plaque might be visible and bad breath might be noticeable.

To confirm the diagnosis, a dental history needs to be taken from the patient, in particular details of their tooth brushing routine. Table 6.3 lists some of the questions that should be asked to aid diagnosis. After questioning, the mouth should be examined.

Conditions to eliminate

Likely causes

Periodontitis Untreated gingivitis can progress to periodontitis. Symptoms are similar to gingivitis but the patient might experience gum bleeding and taste disturbances, and periodontal pockets might be visible. Referral is needed to a dentist for removal of tartar and plaque.

Table 6.3
Specific questions to ask the patient: gingivitis

Question	Relevance
Tooth brushing technique	• Overzealous tooth brushing can lead to bleeding gums and gum recession. Make sure the patient is not 'overcleaning' the teeth
Bleeding gums	• Unprovoked bleeding suggests underlying pathology

Unlikely causes

Medicine–induced gum bleeding Medicines such as warfarin, heparin and non-steroidal anti-inflammatory drugs can produce gum bleeding.

Very unlikely causes

Agranulocytosis and leukaemia Spontaneous bleeding can be a symptom of agranulocytosis or leukaemia. Other symptoms should be present, for example progressive fatigue, weakness and signs of systemic illness such as fever. Urgent referral to the GP is needed.

TRIGGER POINTS indicative of referral: gingivitis

- Foul taste associated with gum bleeding.
- Signs of systemic illness.
- Spontaneous gum bleeding.

Evidence of OTC medicine efficacy

There is no substitute for good oral hygiene. Prevention of plaque build-up by daily brushing is adequate to maintain oral hygiene. Flossing is also recommended to access areas that a toothbrush can miss.

OTC mouthwashes are available but should be reserved for established gingivitis. Mouthwashes containing the anti-bacterial chlorhexidine in concentrations of either 0.1% or 0.2% have proven to be most effective in reducing plaque formation and gingivitis. In clinical trials they have been

> HINTS AND TIPS
>
> ● Discoloration of teeth and tongue: chlorhexidine gluconate
> (e.g. Corsodyl 0.2%, Eludril 0.1%) can stain the tongue and
> teeth brown.

shown to be consistently more effective than placebo and
comparator medicines.

Practical prescribing

Prescribing information relating to mouthwashes is
summarised in the appendix.

Dyspepsia

Dyspepsia is extremely common, and virtually everyone at
some point in their lives will experience symptoms of dyspepsia. OTC management is quite simple; however, healthcare professionals need to ensure symptoms suggestive of
GP intervention are identified.

Arriving at a differential diagnosis

The most likely causes of dyspepsia seen in primary care
are indigestion, heartburn or gastritis. Practitioners should
therefore direct questions to confirm one of these as the
diagnosis as other conditions can cause dyspepsia and are
listed below.

Probability	Cause
Most likely	Indigestion, heartburn or gastritis
Unlikely	Medication, ulcers, irritable bowel syndrome
Very unlikely	Gastric and oesophageal cancers, atypical angina

Clinical features of dyspepsia

Patients with dyspepsia present with a range of symptoms
that commonly involve vague abdominal discomfort
(aching) above the umbilicus and are associated with belching, bloating, flatulence, a feeling of fullness and heartburn.

Although indigestion, heartburn and gastritis will make up the majority of cases presenting in primary care it is important to take a thorough medical and drug history to rule out serious pathology. Table 6.4 lists some of the questions that should be asked to determine the diagnosis.

Table 6.4
Specific questions to ask the patient: dyspepsia

Question	Relevance of question
Age	<ul><li>Young adults are most likely to have dyspepsia</li><li>At > 50 years the chance of underlying pathology increases</li></ul>
Location	<ul><li>Pain above the umbilicus and centrally located (epigastric area) suggests dyspepsia</li><li>Pain below the umbilicus generally suggests lower abdominal conditions such as irritable bowel syndrome, diverticulitis, salpingitis</li><li>Pain experienced behind the sternum (breastbone) suggests heartburn</li><li>Pain that is specific suggests another gastrointestinal condition or even one that is musculoskeletal in origin, e.g. localised renal/biliary colic or muscle strain</li></ul>
Nature of pain	<ul><li>Aching/discomfort suggests dyspepsia</li><li>Gnawing, sharp or stabbing suggests more sinister abdominal pathology, e.g. gastric ulcer</li></ul>
Radiation	<ul><li>Pain that moves from behind the breastbone towards the face or down the left arm suggests a cardiovascular problem</li><li>Pain that moves to the right scapula suggests biliary colic</li><li>Pain that moves to the neck, back or left shoulder suggests angina</li><li>Pain that moves in to the back suggests gastric ulcer</li></ul>

Question	Relevance of question
Severity	<ul><li>Mild/moderate pain suggests non-serious conditions such as dyspepsia</li><li>Severe pain suggests pancreatitis, biliary and renal colic and peritonitis: **refer**</li></ul>
Associated symptoms	<ul><li>Persistent vomiting with or without blood suggests ulcers or even cancer: **refer**</li><li>Black and tarry stools suggest gastrointestinal bleed: **refer**</li></ul>
Aggravating or relieving factors	<ul><li>Pain aggravated by food suggests gastric ulcer: **refer**</li><li>Pain relieved by food suggests duodenal ulcer: **refer**</li></ul>
Social history	<ul><li>Bouts of excessive drinking or eating food too quickly suggest gastritis</li></ul>

Conditions to eliminate

Unlikely causes

Peptic ulceration (gastric and duodenal ulcers)   Typically, the
patient will have well-localised mid-epigastric pain described
as constant, annoying or gnawing. Pain associated with gastric ulcer comes on whenever the stomach is empty, usually
an hour or so after eating, and is generally not relieved by
antacids or food but aggravated by alcohol and caffeine. The
pain of a duodenal ulcer often wakes the patient a few hours
after falling asleep but subsides by morning and is often
relieved after eating. Weight loss and gastrointestinal bleeds
occur more frequently with gastric ulcers.

Medicine-induced dyspepsia   A number of medicines can
cause gastric irritation, leading to or provoking gastrointestinal discomfort:

- aspirin
- ACE inhibitors
- alcohol (in excess)
- iron
- macrolide antibiotics
- metronidazole

- oestrogens
- theophylline.

Irritable bowel syndrome   Upper abdominal pain affects up to a third of patients with irritable bowel syndrome. However, altered defecation – either constipation or diarrhoea with associated bloating – is also normally present. During bouts of diarrhoea mucus tends to be visible on the stools.

Very unlikely causes

Gastric cancer   The patient will usually experience upper abdominal discomfort with nausea and vomiting. Other symptoms associated with carcinoma are gastrointestinal bleeding, fatigue, unexplained weight loss and dysphagia.

Oesophageal cancer   In its early stages, oesophageal cancer can go unnoticed. However, over time the oesophagus becomes constricted and patients will complain of difficulty in swallowing and experience a sensation of food sticking in the oesophagus. As the disease progresses weight loss becomes prominent, despite the patient maintaining a good appetite.

Atypical angina   Not all cases of angina have classic text-book presentation of pain in the retrosternal area with radiation to the neck, back or left shoulder. Patients might complain of dyspepsia-like symptoms and feel generally unwell. These symptoms might be brought on by a heavy meal. In such cases, antacids will fail to relieve symptoms.

Primer for differential diagnosis of dyspepsia

Figure 6.8 helps to aid differentiation of the causes of dyspepsia.

> ## TRIGGER POINTS indicative of referral: dyspepsia
>
> - Dark or tarry stools.
> - Long-standing change in bowel habit.
> - Pain described as severe or debilitating or which wakes the patient in the night.
> - Persistent vomiting (with or without blood).
> - Referred pain.
> - Sensation that food is 'sticking' in the throat.
> - Unexplained weight loss.

Figure 6.8 Primer for differential diagnosis of dyspepsia.

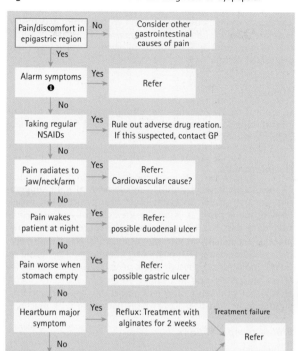

❶ Alarm symptoms. These include, dark stools, persistent vomiting, loss of weight and altered bowel habit.

Evidence of OTC medicine efficacy

Antacids

Antacids have proven efficacy in neutralising stomach acid. However, the neutralising capacity and onset and duration of action of each antacid varies dependent on the metal salt used. Sodium and potassium salts are the most highly soluble, making them quick but short acting. Magnesium and aluminium salts are less soluble and so have a slower onset but greater duration of action. Calcium salts have the advantage of being quick acting yet with a prolonged action. It is therefore commonplace for manufacturers to combine two or more antacid ingredients to ensure a quick onset and prolonged action.

Alginates

In clinical trials, alginate-containing products have demonstrated superior symptom control compared to placebo and antacids for symptoms of heartburn.

H_2 antagonists

There is a paucity of publicly available trial data supporting the use of H_2 antagonists at non-prescription doses. Famotidine appears to have the greatest body of accessible trial data and has been shown to be more effective than placebo and equally as effective as antacids. No trials involving ranitidine using OTC doses on patients could be found on public databases, although trials investigating its inhibitory effect on gastric acid in healthy volunteers showed conclusively that ranitidine, and its comparator drug famotidine, significantly raised intragastric pH compared with placebo.

Proton pump inhibitors

Omeprazole became available over the counter in March 2004. It is marketed under the name Zanprol and licensed for reflux symptoms. Clinical trials have substantiated its efficacy, but it is unclear whether omeprazole is significantly superior to H_2 antagonists or alginates.

HINTS AND TIPS

- Combination products: most antacids are combination products containing two, three or even four constituents. The rationale for combining different salts together appears to be twofold: (i) to ensure that the product has quick onset (containing sodium or calcium) and a long duration of action (containing magnesium, aluminium or calcium); (ii) to counteract each other's side-effect profile.

Practical prescribing

Prescribing information relating to medication for dyspepsia is summarised in the appendix.

Diarrhoea

Diarrhoea is defined as an increase in the frequency of the passage of soft or watery stools relative to the usual bowel habit for that individual. Most patients will self-diagnose diarrhoea, although it is necessary to confirm this because the patient's interpretation of the symptoms might not match up with the medical definition. Diarrhoea can be classed as acute (< 7 days), persistent (> 14 days) or chronic (> 1 month).

Arriving at a differential diagnosis

The most likely cause of diarrhoea seen in primary care is bacterial or viral infection. Practitioners should therefore direct questions to confirm this as other conditions cause diarrhoea and are listed below.

Probability	Cause
Most likely	Viral and bacterial infection
Likely	Medicine induced
Unlikely	Irritable bowel syndrome, giardiasis, faecal impaction
Very unlikely	Ulcerative colitis and Crohn's disease, colorectal cancer, malabsorption syndromes

Clinical features of acute infectious diarrhoea

Symptoms are normally rapid in onset with the patient having a history of prior good health. Nausea and vomiting might be present before or during the bout of acute diarrhoea. Abdominal cramping and tenderness is also often present. If rotavirus is the cause, the patient might also experience viral prodromal symptoms such as cough and cold. Acute infective diarrhoea is usually watery in nature with no blood present. Complete resolution of symptoms should be observed in 2–4 days.

The main priority is identifying those patients who need referral and how quickly they need to be referred. Dehydration is the main complicating factor, especially in the very young and very old. Questions should be aimed at establishing the frequency, fluidity and nature of the stools. Table 6.5 lists some of the questions that should be asked to aid diagnosis.

Table 6.5
Specific questions to ask the patient: diarrhoea

Question	Relevance
Frequency and nature of the stools	• Watery stools in the absence of blood suggest acute infectious diarrhoea • Diarrhoea associated with blood and mucus suggests an invasive infection such as *Shigella* or a condition such as inflammatory bowel disease: **refer**
Periodicity	• A history of recurrent diarrhoea with no identifiable cause should be referred for further investigation: **refer**
Duration	• Chronic diarrhoea should be referred as it suggests irritable bowel syndrome, inflammatory disease or colon cancer: **refer**
Recent food intake	• Eating contaminated food can give rise to symptoms in a matter of a few hours or up to 3 days later • If others ate the same food and are experiencing similar symptoms this suggests food poisoning
Timing of diarrhoea	• Diarrhoea first thing in the morning suggests irritable bowel syndrome • Nocturnal diarrhoea suggests inflammatory bowel disease
Recent travel	• Changes to diet when on holiday can cause changes to bowel function • Travel to a non-Western country increases the chances of people contracting water-borne disease such as giardiasis

Conditions to eliminate

Likely causes

Medicine–induced diarrhoea   A variety of medicines, both POM and OTC, can induce diarrhoea. Some of the more commonly implicated medicines are:

- magnesium-containing antacids
- broad-spectrum antibiotics
- non-steroidal anti-inflammatory drugs
- digoxin at high doses
- excessive alcohol or caffeine ingestion
- proton pump inhibitors
- thiazide diuretics.

Unlikely causes

Giardiasis   The patient will present with watery and foul-smelling diarrhoea accompanied by symptoms of bloating, flatulence and epigastric pain.

Irritable bowel syndrome   The diagnosis is suggested by the presence of long-standing colonic symptoms without any deterioration in the patient's general condition. It is characterised by abdominal pain, especially located in the left lower quadrant of the abdomen. Altered defecation, either constipation or diarrhoea with associated bloating, is also normally present.

Faecal impaction   Faecal impaction is most commonly seen in the elderly. Patients present with continuous soiling as a result of liquid passing around hard stools. Stools are regularly passed but are hard and difficult to pass. Referral is needed.

Very unlikely causes

Ulcerative colitis and Crohn's disease   Both conditions are characterised by periods of remission and relapse. They can affect any age group, although peak incidence is between 20 and 30 years of age. In mild cases, both conditions present with diarrhoea as one of the major symptoms, although blood in the stool is usually present. Patients might also find that they have urgency, nocturnal diarrhoea and early-morning rushes. In the acute phase patients will appear unwell and have malaise.

Malabsorption syndromes Lactose intolerance is often diagnosed in infants under 1 year. In addition to more frequent loose bowel movements, symptoms such as fever, vomiting, perianal excoriation and a failure to gain weight can occur.

Coeliac disease has a bimodal incidence: first, in early infancy, when cereals become a major constituent of the diet, and second between the ages of 40 and 50. Steatorrhoea (fatty stools) is common and can be observed as frothy or floating stools in the toilet pan. Bloating and weight loss in the presence of a normal appetite may also be observed.

Colorectal cancer Any middle-aged patient presenting with a long-standing change of bowel habit must be viewed with suspicion. Persistent diarrhoea accompanied with a feeling that the bowel has not really been emptied is suggestive of neoplasm. This is especially true if weight loss is also present.

Primer for differential diagnosis of diarrhoea

Figure 6.9 helps to aid differentiation of diarrhoeal cases that require referral.

> ### TRIGGER POINTS indicative of referral: diarrhoea
>
> - Change in bowel habit in patients over 50.
> - Diarrhoea following recent travel to tropical or subtropical climate.
> - Duration longer than 2–3 days in children and elderly.
> - Patients unable to drink fluids.
> - Presence of blood or mucus in the stool.
> - Rectal bleeding.
> - Signs of dehydration.
> - Severe abdominal pain.
> - Steatorrhoea.
> - Suspected faecal impaction in the elderly.

Evidence of OTC medicine efficacy

In developed and Western countries, diarrhoeal disease is primarily of economic and socially disruptive significance.

Figure 6.9 Primer for differential diagnosis of diarrhoea.

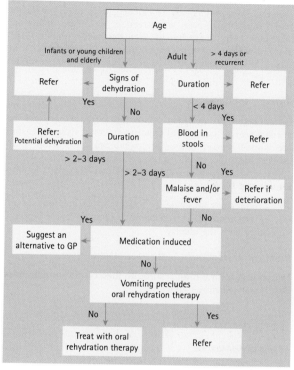

The goals of OTC treatment in the UK are therefore concentrated on relief of symptoms.

Oral rehydration therapy (ORT)

Oral rehydration therapy represents one of the major advances in medicine. It has proven to be a simple, highly effective treatment, which has decreased mortality and morbidity associated with acute diarrhoea in developing countries. More recently, rice-based oral rehydration therapy has begun to be used because in many countries glucose is unavailable. Clinical trials have subsequently shown this to be highly efficacious and well tolerated.

Loperamide

This has been extensively researched, with many published trials investigating its effectiveness in acute infectious diarrhoea. The majority of well-designed, double-blind, placebo-controlled trials have consistently shown it to be significantly better than placebo and comparable to diphe-noxylate (Lomotil).

Bismuth subsalicylate

Bismuth-containing products are now infrequently used but are superior to placebo in treating traveller's diarrhoea but are significantly slower in symptom resolution than loperamide.

Kaolin and morphine

This product has no evidence to support its use and should not be recommended. It remains a popular home remedy, especially with the elderly.

Practical prescribing

Prescribing information relating to medication for diarrhoea is summarised in the appendix.

110

HINTS AND TIPS

Signs of dehydration
- Mild (< 5%) dehydration is characterised by slightly dry mucous membranes, loss of skin turgor and sunken eyes.
- Moderate (5–10%) dehydration is characterised by a sunken fontanelle (in infants) and eyes, dry mouth and decreased urine output; the patient will be moderately thirsty.

Constipation

Constipation, like diarrhoea, means different things to different people. It can be defined as a reduction in the number of stools passed (to that person) and accompanied by more difficult defecation and/or hard stools. Constipation is extremely common and occurs in all age groups but is especially prevalent in the elderly.

Arriving at a differential diagnosis

The most likely cause of constipation seen in primary care in all ages is related to social factors. Practitioners should therefore direct questions to confirm this as other conditions cause constipation and are listed below.

Probability	Cause
Most likely	Eating habits, lifestyle
Likely	Medication
Unlikely	Irritable bowel syndrome, pregnancy, depression, functional disorders (children)
Very unlikely	Colorectal cancer, hypothyroidism

Clinical features of constipation

As well as problems associated with defecation, patients may have abdominal discomfort and bloating. A child's parents might also notice that the child is more irritable than normal and has a decreased appetite. Specks of blood in the toilet pan may be present and are usually the result of straining at stool.

111

Constipation is rarely caused by sinister pathology. Table 6.6 lists some of the questions that should be asked to aid diagnosis and decide if referral to a GP is needed.

Conditions to eliminate

Likely causes

Medicine-induced constipation Many medicines can cause constipation; some are more commonly implicated than others:

- anticholinergics, e.g. TCAs, antiparkinsonian drugs, antipsychotics
- antihypertensives, e.g. verapamil
- opiate analgesics
- aluminium-containing antacids
- iron
- sucralfate (contains aluminium).

Table 6.6
Specific questions to ask the patient: constipation

Question	Relevance
Who is the patient?	• Constipation in adults usually stems from a social/lifestyle problem • In children there is often a behavioural cause
Pain on defecation	• Pain on defecation suggests a local anorectal problem (e.g. anal fissure) • Children who experience pain on defecation might suppress defecation and thus exacerbate the constipation
Presence of blood	• Bright-red specks in the toilet or smears on toilet tissue suggest haemorrhoids or a tear in the anal fissure • Blood is mixed in the stool (melaena) suggests a gastrointestinal bleed: **refer**
Duration	• Long-standing constipation (> 14 days) with no identifiable cause or previous investigation by the GP suggests underlying pathology: **refer**
Social circumstances	• Changes in job or marital status can precipitate depressive illness that can manifest with symptoms such as constipation

Unlikely causes

Irritable bowel syndrome The diagnosis is suggested by the presence of long-standing colonic symptoms without any deterioration in the patient's general condition. It is characterised by abdominal pain, especially in the left (or sometimes the right) lower quadrant of the abdomen. Altered defecation, either constipation or diarrhoea, with associated bloating is also normally present.

Pregnancy Constipation is common in the third trimester, and most patients complain of hard stools rather than a decrease in bowel movements. A combination of factors, including increased circulating progestogen, displacement of the uterus against the colon and iron supplementation, all contribute to an increased incidence of constipation.

Functional causes in children The causes of constipation in children are various and normally result from a traumatic experience associated with defecation, e.g. pain when going to the toilet.

Depression It is reported that a third of patients suffering from depression present with gastrointestinal symptoms, often constipation. Healthcare practitioners should therefore be mindful of this and make appropriate checks for precipitating factors or symptoms that suggest depression.

Very unlikely causes

Colorectal cancer Colorectal carcinomas are rare in patients under the age of 40. The patient might complain of abdominal pain, rectal bleeding and tenesmus. Weight loss – a classic textbook sign of colon cancer – is common but observed only in the later stages of the disease.

Hypothyroidism The symptoms of hypothyroidism are often subtle and insidious in onset. As well as constipation, patients might experience weight gain, lethargy, coarse hair and dry skin.

113

Primer for differential diagnosis of constipation

Figure 6.10 helps aid differentiation between common and more serious causes of constipation.

> **! TRIGGER POINTS indicative of referral: constipation**
>
> - Duration more than 14 days with no identifiable cause.
> - Pain on defecation causing patient to suppress the defecatory reflex.
> - Patients aged over 40 years old with sudden change in bowel habits with no obvious cause.
> - Suspected depression.

Figure 6.10 Primer for differential diagnosis of constipation.

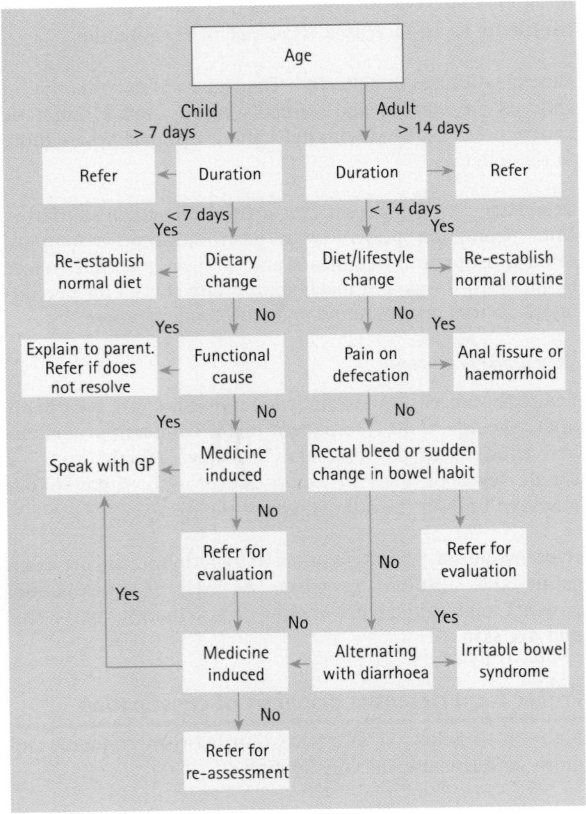

Evidence of OTC medicine efficacy

Increasing dietary fibre and fluid intake as well as more exercise will relieve the majority of acute cases of constipation. If medication is required, all four classes of OTC laxative (stimulant, osmotic, bulk-forming and stool softeners) have evidence of efficacy, although as yet no trials have determined if one class of laxative is superior to another. Choice of laxative will therefore be driven by patient need and acceptability.

HINTS AND TIPS

Onset of action

- Bulk-forming laxatives (e.g. ispaghula husk, methylcellulose and sterculia): can take up to 72 hours to take effect.
- Osmotic laxatives (e.g. magnesium salts and lactulose): can take from 3 hours (magnesium) to > 24 hours (lactulose) to take effect.
- Stimulant laxatives (e.g. senna, bisacodyl, sodium picosulfate): can take 6–12 hours to take effect.
- Stool softeners (e.g. docusate): can take 6–12 hours to take effect.

Administration

- Each methylcellulose (Celevac) tablet should be taken with at least 300 mL of liquid.
- Sterculia (Normacol and Normacol Plus granules or sachets): the granules should be placed dry on the tongue and swallowed immediately with plenty of water or a cool drink. They can also be sprinkled onto and taken with soft food such as yoghurt.

Pregnancy

If a laxative is required, a bulk-forming laxative should be recommended.

Administration of suppositories: instructions to the patient

1. Wash your hands.
2. Lie on one side with your knees pulled up towards your chest.
3. Gently push the suppository, pointed end first, into your back passage with your finger. Push the suppository in as far as possible.
4. Lower your legs, roll over onto your stomach and remain still for a few minutes.
5. If you feel your body trying to expel the suppository, try to resist this. Lie still and press your buttocks together.
6. Wash your hands.

115

Practical prescribing

Prescribing information relating to medication for constipation is summarised in the appendix.

Haemorrhoids

Haemorrhoids (piles) can occur in patients of any age but are more common in people aged between 40 and 65 and in pregnant women; they are rare in patients aged under 20. Patients might feel embarrassed talking about symptoms and it is therefore important that any requests for advice are treated sympathetically and away from others to avoid embarrassment.

Arriving at a differential diagnosis

The most likely cause of anal irritation/pain seen in primary care is haemorrhoids. Practitioners should therefore direct questions to confirm this diagnosis as other conditions can cause pain/irritation and are listed below.

Probability	Cause
Most likely	Prolapsed haemorrhoids
Likely	Anal fissure
Unlikely	Dermatitis
Very unlikely	Colorectal cancer, inflammatory bowel disease, upper gastrointestinal bleeds

Clinical features of haemorrhoids

Bleeding, pain and perianal itching can all occur but patients might be asymptomatic until the haemorrhoid prolapses. After defecation, the haemorrhoids might spontaneously return to their normal position or be reduced manually. Blood is bright red and is most commonly seen as spotting around the toilet pan, streaking on toilet tissue or visible on the surface of the stool. Pain is often described as a dull ache that increases in severity when the patient defecates. This can make the patient ignore the urge to defecate, resulting in constipation, which in turn will lead to more difficulty in passing stools and increase the pain associated with defecation.

Bleeding tends to cause the greatest concern and often instigates the patient to seek help. Table 6.7 lists some of the

Table 6.7
Specific questions to ask the patient: haemorrhoids

Question	Relevance
Duration	• Patients with haemorrhoids tend to have had symptoms for some time before requesting advice. Patients with symptoms that have been present for > 3 weeks should be referred
Pain	• A dull aching pain not necessarily related to defecation (e.g. when sitting) suggests haemorrhoids • Sharp or stabbing pain at the time of defecation suggests an anal fissure or tear
Rectal bleeding	• Slight rectal bleeding that is bright red suggests haemorrhoids • Blood mixed in the stool suggests a gastrointestinal bleed • Blood loss not associated with defecation suggests carcinoma
Associated symptoms	• Localised anal itching suggests haemorrhoids or dermatitis • Nausea, vomiting, loss of appetite and altered bowel habit suggests sinister pathology: **refer**

117

questions that should be asked to help diagnosis and eliminate more sinister pathology.

Conditions to eliminate

Likely causes

Anal fissure   Straining at stool can cause anal fissures. Pain can be intense and blood, if passed, is bright red. Non-urgent referral is necessary for confirmation of the diagnosis. In the meantime, patients should be instructed to eat more fibre and to increase their intake of fluids.

Unlikely causes

Dermatitis If pruritus is the chief presenting symptom and the patient does not complain of bleeding or prolapse then dermatitis caused by toiletries or scratching should be considered.

Very unlikely causes (conditions causing rectal bleeding)

Ulcerative colitis and Crohn's disease Other symptoms besides blood in the stool are usually present. These tend to be watery stools, abdominal pain and fever. Patients will appear unwell and have urgency, nocturnal diarrhoea and early morning rushes. In the acute phase patients will have malaise.

Upper gastrointestinal bleeds Gastrointestinal bleeds are often associated with non-steroidal anti-inflammatory drug intake. The colour of the stool is related to the rate of bleeding. Stools from gastrointestinal bleeds can be tarry (indicating a bleed of 100–200 mL of blood) or black (indicating a bleed of 400–500 mL of blood). Urgent referral is needed.

Colorectal cancer A change of bowel habit in any middle-aged patient, especially if long established, must be viewed with suspicion. Colorectal bleeds depend on the site of tumour, for example sigmoid tumours, lead to bright-red blood in or around the stool. Rectal bleeding tends to be persistent and steady, though slight, for all tumours.

Primer for differential diagnosis of haemorrhoids

Figure 6.11 helps aid differentiation of haemorrhoids.

> **TRIGGER POINTS indicative of referral: haemorrhoids**
>
> - Abdominal pain.
> - Blood in the stool.
> - Fever.
> - Patients who have to manually reduce their haemorrhoids.
> - Persistent change in bowel habit in middle-aged patients.
> - Unexplained rectal bleeding.

Figure 6.11   Primer for differential diagnosis of haemorrhoids.

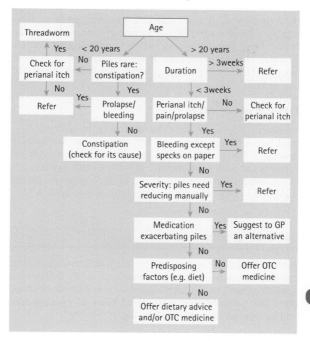

Evidence of OTC medicine efficacy

Numerous products are marketed for the relief and treatment of haemorrhoids. These include a wide range of therapeutic agents and commonly include anaesthetics, astringents, anti-inflammatories and protectorants. Most products contain a combination of these agents, with some having three or more different agents included. The inclusion of such a diverse range of chemical entities appears to be based largely on theoretical grounds rather than any evidence base. Extensive literature searching found only one published trial regarding the efficacy of any marketed product. However, this trial suffered from serious methodological flaws. With so few data available on their effectiveness it is impossible to say whether any product is a credible treatment for haemorrhoids, and many medical authorities regard them as little more than placebos. However, products containing a local anaesthetic or hydrocortisone will probably confer some benefit because of their proven effectiveness in other, similar, conditions. It would therefore seem most prudent if recommending a product that it should contain one or both of these chemical entities.

Practical prescribing

Treatment should be recommended only to patients with mild haemorrhoids. If manual reduction of haemorrhoids is necessary, the patient should be referred for non-surgical intervention with sclerotherapy or rubber band ligation.

Prescribing information relating to medication for haemorrhoids is summarised in the appendix and in Table 6.8.

Abdominal pain

Abdominal pain is a symptom of many different conditions ranging from acute self-limiting problems to life-threatening conditions such as ruptured appendicitis and bowel obstruction. The overwhelming majority of cases in primary care will be non-serious and self-limiting.

Arriving at a differential diagnosis

The most likely causes of abdominal pain will be dyspepsia, irritable bowel syndrome and gastroenteritis. Practitioners should therefore direct questions to establish if one of these conditions is responsible for the patient's symptoms as many other causes of abdominal pain are seen in primary care; these are listed below.

Clinical features of dyspepsia

Patients with dyspepsia present with a range of symptoms that commonly involve vague abdominal discomfort (aching) above the umbilicus that is associated with belching, bloating, flatulence, a feeling of fullness and heartburn. It is normally relieved by antacids and aggravated by spicy foods or excessive caffeine; vomiting is unusual.

Table 6.8
Practical prescribing:
summary of haemorrhoid products

	Form	Anaesthetic	Astringent	Steroid	Protectorant
Anacal*	Cream or suppository	No	No	No	No
Anodesyn	Ointment or suppository	Yes	No	No	No
Anusol	Cream, ointment or suppository	No	Yes	No	No
Anusol Plus	Ointment or suppository	No	Yes	Yes	No
Germoloids	Cream, ointment or suppository	Yes	Yes	No	No
Germoloids HC	Spray	Yes	No	Yes	No
Hemocane	Cream	Yes	No	No	No
Nupercainal	Ointment	Yes	No	No	No
Perinal	Spray	Yes	No	Yes	No
Preparation H	Ointment or suppository	No	No	No	Yes

*Contains a sclerosing agent.

121

Probability	Cause		
	Upper abdomen	*Lower abdomen*	*Diffuse*
Most likely	Dyspepsia	Irritable bowel syndrome	Gastroenteritis
Likely	Peptic ulcers	Diverticulitis (elderly)	Not applicable
Unlikely	Cholecystitis, cholelithiasis, renal colic	Appendicitis, endometriosis, renal colic	Not applicable
Very unlikely	Splenic enlargement, hepatitis, myocardial infarction	Ectopic pregnancy, salpingitis, intestinal obstruction	Pancreatitis, peritonitis

Clinical features of irritable bowel syndrome (IBS)

The diagnosis is suggested by the presence of long-standing colonic symptoms without any deterioration in the patient's general condition. Irritable bowel syndrome is characterised by abdominal pain, especially located in the left (or sometimes the right) lower quadrant of the abdomen. Altered defecation, either constipation or diarrhoea, with associated bloating is also normally present.

Clinical features of gastroenteritis

Symptoms of nausea, vomiting and diarrhoea will generally be more prominent than abdominal pain. The patient might also have a fever and suffer from general malaise.

In abdominal pain, single symptoms are poor predictors of final diagnosis (except heartburn in reflux oesophagitis). It is therefore important to use knowledge on the incidence and prevalence of conditions to determine if referral is needed. In addition, the location of the pain is helpful to narrow down the cause of the pain, as certain conditions will give rise to symptoms in certain parts of the abdomen. Table 6.9 lists the questions that should be asked to aid diagnosis.

Table 6.9
Specific questions to ask the patient: abdominal pain

Question	Relevance
Nature of the pain	• A retrosternal burning sensation is highly suggestive of heartburn • Cramp-like pain suggests diverticulitis, irritable bowel syndrome, salpingitis and gastroenteritis • Colicky pain suggests appendicitis, biliary and renal colic and intestinal obstruction
Radiating pain (abdominal pain that moves from its original site should be viewed with caution)	• Pain that radiates to the jaw, face and arm suggests cardiovascular origin • Pain that moves from a central location to the right lower quadrant suggests appendicitis • Pain radiating to the back suggests peptic ulcer or pancreatitis
Severity of pain	• Mild/moderate pain suggests non-serious conditions • Severe pain suggests pancreatitis, biliary and renal colic and peritonitis
Age of patient	• Increasing age increases the likelihood of an identifiable and serious organic cause • Appendicitis is the only serious abdominal condition that is more common in the young
Onset of pain	• Sudden onset suggests a more serious condition, e.g. peritonitis, appendicitis, ectopic pregnancy, renal and biliary colic
Aggravating/relieving factors	• Pain not eased with antacids suggests gastric ulcer • Pain worsened by food suggests gastric ulcer or biliary colic • Pain worsened by movement suggests salpingitis, pancreatitis and appendicitis

123

Conditions to eliminate: upper abdomen

Likely causes

Peptic ulcer (gastric and duodenal) These occur most commonly in patients aged 30–50 years. Typically, pain is epigastric and described as constant, annoying or gnawing. In gastric ulcers, pain comes on whenever the stomach is empty, usually an hour or so after eating, and is generally relieved by antacids or food but aggravated by alcohol and caffeine. Pain in duodenal ulcers tends to wake the person at night.

Unlikely causes

Acute cholecystitis and cholelithiasis Acute cholecystitis (inflammation of the gall bladder) and cholelithiasis (presence of gallstones in the bile ducts, also called biliary colic) are characterised by persistent, steady, severe, aching pain. Onset is sudden and starts a few hours after a meal, frequently waking the patient in the early hours of the morning. The pain might radiate to the tip of the right scapula in cholelithiasis. Fatty foods often aggravate the pain.

Renal colic (stones) Stones most frequently get lodged in the ureter. Pain begins in the loin, radiating round the flank into the groin and sometimes down the inner side of the thigh. Pain is severe and colicky and attacks tend to last hours. Nausea and vomiting might also be present.

Very unlikely causes

Splenic enlargement or rupture
Generalised left upper quadrant pain associated with abdominal fullness and early feeding satiety is observed. The condition is nearly always secondary to another primary cause, which could be an infection, the result of inflammation or haematological.

Hepatitis Liver enlargement from any type of hepatitis will cause discomfort or dull pain. Associated symptoms of nausea, vomiting, jaundice and pruritus should be present.

Myocardial ischaemia Angina and myocardial infarction cause chest pain that might initially be difficult to distinguish from dyspepsia. Cardiovascular pain often radiates to the neck, jaw and inner aspect of the left arm. Typically, angina pain is precipitated by exertion and subsides after a few minutes once at rest. The patient might appear pale, display weakness and be tachycardic.

Conditions to eliminate: lower abdomen

Likely causes

Diverticulitis   This is most prevalent in the elderly and is characterised by cramp-like pain in the left lower quadrant, although the pain can also be suprapubic and occasionally in the right lower quadrant. Fever is a prominent feature and the patient generally has a history of constipation and diarrhoea.

Appendicitis   Classically the pain starts in the mid-abdomen around the umbilicus before moving to the right lower quadrant, although right-sided pain is experienced from the outset in about 50% of patients. Pain is described as colicky or cramp like that becomes constant. Movement tends to aggravate the pain and vomiting might also be present.

Unlikely causes

Renal colic (stones)   Stones most frequently get lodged in the ureter. Pain begins in the loin radiating round the flank into the groin and sometimes down the inner side of the thigh. Pain is severe and colicky and attacks tend to last hours. Symptoms of nausea and vomiting may also be present.

Endometriosis   Patients experience lower abdominal aching pain that can be constant and severe. Symptoms usually start 5–7 days before menstruation and often worsen at the onset of bleeding. Pain into the back and down the thighs is also possible.

Very unlikely causes

Intestinal obstruction   Intestinal obstruction has sudden and acute onset. The pain is described as colicky and can be experienced anywhere in the lower abdomen. Constipation and vomiting are prominent features.

Ectopic pregnancy   Patients suffer from persistent moderate to severe pain that is sudden in onset. A menstrual history will reveal that the patient's last period is late.

Salpingitis (inflammation of the fallopian tubes) Predominantly, salpingitis occurs in young sexually active women, especially those fitted with an intrauterine device. Pain is usually bilateral and cramping and starts shortly after menstruation.

Conditions to eliminate: diffuse

Very unlikely causes

Pancreatitis Pain of pancreatitis develops suddenly and is described as agonising, with the pain being centrally located and often radiating into the back. The pain reaches its maximum intensity within minutes and can last hours or days. Vomiting is common but does not relieve the pain. It is commonly seen in alcoholics.

Peritonitis Although the pain of acute peritonitis can be diffuse, severe pain in the upper abdomen is often present. This is accompanied by intense rigidity of the abdominal wall producing a 'board-like' appearance. Vomiting might also be present.

Primer for differential diagnosis of abdominal pain

126

Figure 6.12 helps aid differentiation of abdominal pain.

> **!** **TRIGGER POINTS indicative of referral: abdominal pain**
>
> - Abdominal pain not relieved by vomiting.
> - Abdominal pain with fever.
> - Elderly.
> - Haematemesis.
> - Melaena.
> - Pregnancy.
> - Trauma.
> - Severe pain or pain that radiates.

Evidence of OTC medicine efficacy for dyspepsia

Antacids, alginates, H_2 antagonists and proton pump inhibitors are all effective in controlling dyspepsia symptoms. Alginates should be used first line for heartburn

Figure 6.12   Primer for differential diagnosis of abdominal pain.

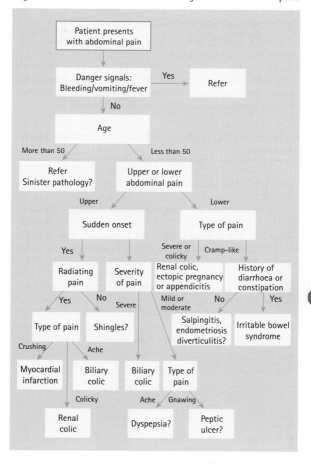

127

symptoms but for more generalised and non-specific symptoms either an antacid or H_2 antagonist could be tried, as both classes of medicine have proven efficacy and appear to be clinically equivalent. Proton pump inhibitors may be a useful alternative for those patients who have recurrent attacks.

Evidence of OTC medicine efficacy for gastroenteritis

Oral rehydration therapy (ORT)

Of greatest significance is fluid loss associated with gastroenteritis, especially in the young and elderly. Oral rehydration therapy is a highly effective treatment in returning electrolyte balance to normal and should be recommended as first-line treatment if diarrhoea and vomiting are present. For pain, simple analgesia can be recommended.

Evidence of OTC medicine efficacy for irritable bowel syndrome

OTC medicines for the treatment of the symptoms irritable bowel syndrome include hyoscine, mebeverine and peppermint oil.

Only mebeverine has reasonable trial data to support its efficacy. A meta-analysis by Poynard (*Alimentary Pharmacology and Therapeutics* 2001; 15: 355–361) that included non-English language papers suggests that there is a significant difference between mebeverine and placebo. Pittler et al (*American Journal of Gastroenterology* 1998; 93: 1375–1381) reviewed papers involving peppermint oil and concluded that study design limitations meant that definitive judgement about efficacy was not possible, although it could be efficacious for symptom relief. Trials involving hyoscine have shown it to be no better than placebo.

Chapter 7

Dermatology

The skin is the largest organ of the body and performs many important functions. These include barring entry to micro-organisms, acting as a sensory organ (e.g. for pressure or pain), regulating body temperature and maintaining the body's homeostatic balance.

History taking

With most skin conditions a number of general questions should always be asked. Table 7.1 highlights these questions.

Physical examination

A more accurate differential diagnosis will be made if the 'rash' is examined, as patient descriptions of rashes will be variable. Asking to see the rash/condition enables the healthcare practitioner to base the differential diagnosis on more than just questioning. Examination should be possible in the majority of cases, providing there is adequate privacy. Table 7.2 highlights a number of things to look for when examining a patient.

Acne vulgaris

Acne affects virtually all adolescents. The peak incidence is 14–17 years for girls and 15–19 years for boys. Acne usually resolves within 10 years of onset, although women in their 30s can have mild persistent acne.

Arriving at a differential diagnosis

Diagnosis is straightforward and most patients will generally be seeking appropriate advice on correct product selection. However, a few conditions can present with acne-like lesions and need to be excluded; these are listed below.

Probability	Cause
Most likely	Mild acne
Likely	Rosacea, moderate/severe acne
Unlikely	Medicine-induced acne

Table 7.1
Questions to consider when taking a dermatological history

Question	Relevance
Where did the problem first appear?	Certain skin problems start in one particular location before spreading to other parts of the body, e.g. impetigo usually starts on the face before spreading to the limbs
Are there any other symptoms?	Most conditions exhibit itch and/or pain, e.g. mild itch is associated with psoriasis and medicine eruptions; severe itch is associated with scabies, atopic and contact dermatitis
Occupational history (relevant to adults only)	In some occupations workers are exposed to irritants and chemicals, e.g. hairdressing
General medical history	Skin defects might be the first sign of internal disease, e.g. diabetes can manifest with pruritus and thyroid disease can present with hair loss and pruritus
Foreign travel	Tropical skin conditions can be contracted when abroad but lesions do not appear until the person has returned home
Family and household contact history	Some skin disorders, such as scabies, can infect those with whom the patient is in close contact
The patient's thoughts on the cause of the problem	Ask for the patient's opinion. This might help with the diagnosis or shed light on anxieties

Table 7.2
Performing a dermatological examination

Lesions	Relevance
Temperature	• Using the backs of your fingers you should be able to identify generalised warmth or coolness of the skin, e.g. generalised warmth might indicate fever, whereas local warmth could indicate inflammation or cellulitis
Distribution	• Look at the pattern of involvement of the skin. Many skin diseases have a 'typical' or 'classic' distribution • Psoriasis typically affects elbows, knees, scalp and the sacral areas • Adult seborrhoeic dermatitis affects the face and mid-chest
Lesion shape	• Are the lesions arciform (in an arc), linear, annular (in a ring) or clustered, e.g. tinea corporis (ringworm) infection usually presents as an annular rash?
Recent trauma	• Have the lesions developed on a site of trauma or injury? This is seen in a number of conditions such as psoriasis and warts
Touching the skin	• Do not be afraid to touch a patient's skin; very few skin conditions are infectious

131

Clinical features of mild acne vulgaris

Patients suffering from mild acne predominantly have open and closed comedones (blackheads and whiteheads) with a small number of active lesions normally confined to the face.

Differential diagnosis of acne is routine but an assessment of the severity is required. Most dermatology books simply grade the severity of acne in to mild, moderate or severe. Table 7.3 lists some of the questions that should be asked to help determine severity and if referral is needed.

Table 7.3
Specific questions to ask the patient: acne vulgaris

Question	Relevance
Severity	● Moderate acne is not confined to the face but also involves the back and chest. Lesions are often painful and there is a real possibility of scarring ● Severe acne has all the characteristics of moderate acne plus the development of cysts. Lesions are often widespread and scarring is frequent
Age of onset	● Patients with acne-like lesions who are outside the normal age range suggest an adverse drug reaction or rosacea
Occupation	● Certain jobs can predispose patients to acne-like lesions, e.g. car mechanics exposed to long-term contact with oils

Conditions to eliminate

Likely causes

Rosacea   Normally seen in patients over 40 years of age, rosacea is classically characterised by acne-like lesions and recurrent flushing of the central face, especially the nose and medial cheeks. Eye irritation and blepharitis also occurs in up to 20% of patients.

Moderate/severe acne   Widespread facial lesions and involvement on the chest and back should be referred for topical or systemic antibiotic treatment or vitamin A derivatives.

Unlikely causes

Medicines causing acne-like skin eruptions   A number of medicines can produce acne-like lesions:

● lithium
● oral contraceptives (especially those with high progestogen levels)
● phenytoin

- azathioprine
- rifampicin.

TRIGGER POINTS indicative of referral: acne vulgaris

- Moderate or severe acne.
- Occupational acne.
- OTC treatment failure.
- Rosacea.

Evidence of OTC medicine efficacy

OTC acne treatments contain benzoyl peroxide, salicylic acid, sulphur or an antibacterial. Benzoyl peroxide has the greatest body of evidence to support its use. Many studies have proved the efficacy of benzoyl peroxide in mild to moderate acne. Owing to its potential to cause erythema and irritation, concentrations of 10% are probably best avoided, especially as 5% and 10% concentrations seem to be equally efficacious. A variety of other agents (e.g. miconazole and hydrocortisone) have been used in combination with benzoyl peroxide but none has proved to be significantly better than benzoyl peroxide alone.

Salicylic acid and sulphur have been used for many years on the basis of their keratolytic action but based on evidence they are probably best avoided.

133

HINTS AND TIPS

- Length of treatment: approximately 60% of patients should see an improvement in their symptoms after 8–12 weeks. If symptoms fail to improve after this time then referral to a GP would be appropriate.
- Benzoyl peroxide: benzoyl peroxide can cause drying, burning and peeling on initial application. If patients experience these side-effects then they should be told to stop using the product for a day or two before starting again. Patients should therefore start on the lowest strength commercially available, especially if they suffer from sensitive or fair skin.

Practical prescribing

Prescribing information relating to acne medication is summarised in the appendix.

Cold sores

Cold sores are caused by the herpes simplex virus. Infection most often results from direct contact of mucous membranes (e.g. kissing) or contact at sites of abraded skin between an infected and an uninfected individual. The virus then infects epidermal and dermal cells, causing skin vesicles.

Arriving at a differential diagnosis

The most likely cause of a sore on the outside of the mouth encountered in primary care is an infection by herpes simplex. Practitioners should therefore direct questions to confirm this diagnosis as other conditions give rise to similar symptoms and are listed below.

Probability	Cause
Most likely	Cold sore
Likely	Impetigo
Unlikely	Angular cheilitis

134

Clinical features of cold sores

Patients with cold sores generally experience itching, burning or tingling symptoms from a few hours to a couple of days before the eruption of lesions. The lesions appear as blisters and vesicles with associated redness (Fig. 7.1). The blisters then crust over, usually within 24 hours, and tend to itch and be painful. The lesions spontaneously resolve in 7–10 days. Many patients can identify a cause of their cold sore, with sunlight (ultraviolet light) reported to induce cold sores in 20% of sufferers. Recurrence is common and patients will often experience two or three episodes each year.

Cold sores should not be too difficult to diagnose but a number of questions should be asked to confirm the diagnosis (Table 7.4).

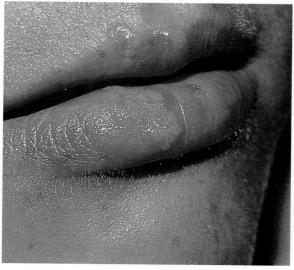

Figure 7.1 Cold sore. Reproduced from *Color Atlas of Dermatology* by G White, 2004, Churchill Livingstone, with permission.

Conditions to eliminate

Likely causes

Impetigo Impetigo usually starts as a small red itchy patch of inflamed skin that quickly develops into vesicles that rupture and weep (Fig. 7.2). The exudate dries to a brown–yellow, sticky crust. It is contagious and children should be kept away from school until the rash clears. Not sharing towels will help to stop household contacts contracting the infection.

Unlikely causes

Angular cheilitis Angular cheilitis can occur at any age but is more common in the elderly, especially those who wear dentures. The corners of the mouth become cracked, fissured and red. The lesions can become boggy and macerated, and are slow to heal as movement of the mouth hinders healing. It is painful but generally does not itch or crust over.

Table 7.4
Specific questions to ask the patient: cold sores

Question	Relevance
Appearance	• 'Warning' symptoms before the skin eruption suggests a cold sore • A yellow, crusty lesion with no warning symptoms suggests impetigo • Lesions that crack and fissure suggest angular cheilitis
Location	• Lesions on the mouth suggest cold sores (but they might also occur around and inside the nose, but this is less common) • A rash that spreads to other areas of the face or body suggests impetigo • A lesion just at the corners of the mouth suggests angular cheilitis
Trigger factors	• Stress, ill health and sunlight are all implicated in triggering cold sore attacks. These triggers are not seen with other similar conditions

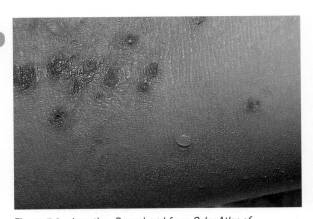

Figure 7.2 Impetigo. Reproduced from *Color Atlas of Dermatology* by G White, 2004, Churchill Livingstone, with permission.

TRIGGER POINTS indicative of referral: cold sores

- Duration > 14 days.
- Lesions within the mouth.
- Lesions that spread rapidly over the face.
- Patients who take immunosuppressive medicines.
- Severe and widespread lesions.
- Systemic symptoms such as fever and malaise.

Evidence of OTC medicine efficacy

A number of OTC products are marketed for the relief and treatment of cold sores. None has been shown conclusively to be effective in prevention or treatment. Products containing ammonia, zinc and povidone iodine appear to have no evidence of efficacy. Only topical aciclovir has demonstrated some clinical effectiveness. Trial data support its use as a prophylactic agent if applied in the prodromal stage and total healing time is reduced by approximately 24 hours. Other products containing local anaesthetics and analgesics might be of value to reduce the pain and itching associated with cold sores.

Practical prescribing

Prescribing information relating to medication for cold sores is summarised in the appendix.

Corns and calluses

A combination of friction and pressure over a prolonged period of time causes corn and callus formation.

Arriving at a differential diagnosis

The most likely cause of corns and calluses is inappropriate footwear. Practitioners should therefore direct questions to confirm this as the cause as other conditions can give rise to similar symptoms.

Probability	Cause
Most likely	Corns and calluses caused from footwear
Likely	Verruca
Unlikely	Bunions

Clinical features of corns

Corns are either soft or hard. Hard corns are generally located on the tops of the toes whereas soft corns form between the toes. A hard corn appears as a painful raised yellow ring of inflammatory skin with a central core of hard grey skin. Soft corns appear white and remain soft due to moisture causing maceration of the corn. Soft corns are most common in the fourth web space.

Clinical features of calluses

Calluses, depending on the cause and site involved, can range in size from a few millimetres to centimetres. They appear as flattened, yellowish-white and thickened skin. The balls of the feet, heel and lower border of the big toe are common sites. Patients frequently complain of a burning sensation resulting from fissuring of the callus.

Differential diagnosis should be simple. Table 7.5 lists some of the questions that will help to determine the best course of action.

Conditions to eliminate

Likely causes

Verrucas Verrucas tend to have a spongy texture with the central area showing tiny black spots. They are rarely located on or between the toes and commonly occur in patients younger than those who experience corns and calluses.

Unlikely causes

Bunions Bunions are more common in women than men. Initially, irritation of skin by ill-fitting shoes causes bursitis of the big toe. Over time, the inflamed area solidifies into a gelatinous mass resulting in a bunion joint. This will be seen

Table 7.5
**Specific questions to ask the patient:
corns and calluses**

Question	Relevance
Location	● Lesions on the tops or between toes suggest a corn ● A lesion on the plantar surface of the foot suggests a verruca
Aggravating or relieving factors	● Pain relieved by removing footwear suggests a corn ● Pain with or without footwear suggests a verruca
Appearance	● A white or yellow hyperkeratinised area of skin suggests a corn or callus ● Black 'dots' on the surface of the lesion suggest a verruca

as a lump on the instep of the foot just below the big toe. Referral is needed.

TRIGGER POINTS indicative of referral: corns and calluses

● Discomfort/pain causing difficulty walking.
● Soft corns.
● Treatment failure.

139

Evidence of OTC medicine efficacy

Corns and calluses are due to friction and pressure. Removal of the precipitating factors and preventative measures form the mainstay of treatment. Correctly fitting shoes are essential to help prevent their formation. If pressure and friction still persist when correctly fitted shoes are worn then patients might obtain relief by shielding or padding. Moleskin or thin podiatry felt placed around the corn allows pressure to be transferred from the corn to the padding. In callus formation a 'shock-absorbing' insert such as a metatarsal pad is useful to relieve weight on the callus and so reduce stress on the plantar skin. Treatment should be avoided if possible, but if deemed appropriate keratolytics can be used, although there is no evidence to suggest that they are effective.

Practical prescribing

Prescribing information relating to medication for corns and calluses is summarised in the appendix.

HINTS AND TIPS

A number of proprietary products are specifically marketed for the relief of corns and calluses, e.g. products in the Carnation and Scholl range (medicated and non-medicated corn pads, callous foam cushions, bunion guards, etc.). A full listing can be obtained from the *Chemist and Druggist* monthly price list that is kept in virtually all pharmacies.

Dandruff (pityriasis capitis)

Dandruff is very common, affecting all ages and either sex. It is a chronic relapsing non-inflammatory hyperproliferative skin condition resulting from increased cell turnover rate.

Arriving at a differential diagnosis

The most likely scalp condition to be encountered in primary care is dandruff, although a number of conditions need to be eliminated and are listed below.

Probability	Cause
Most likely	Pityriasis capitis (dandruff)
Likely	Contact dermatitis, scalp psoriasis (mild)
Unlikely	Seborrhoeic dermatitis
Very unlikely	Tinea capitis

Clinical features of dandruff

The scalp will be dry, itchy and flaky. Often, visible dead cells can be seen on the clothing. Most patients will diagnose and treat dandruff without seeking medical help. If advice is sought then Table 7.6 lists the questions that should be asked to aid the diagnosis.

Conditions to eliminate

Likely causes

Contact dermatitis   The use of new hair products such as dyes and perms can result in irritation and scaling. Avoidance of the irritant should see an improvement in the condition. If improvement is not observed after 1–2 weeks then reassessment is needed.

Mild scalp psoriasis   In mild scalp psoriasis, redness and scaling might be less prominent or even absent. However, the rash still tends to show clear demarcation, which should allow differentiation from dandruff.

Unlikely causes

Seborrhoeic dermatitis   Typically seborrhoeic dermatitis will affect areas other than the scalp. In adults, the trunk is

Table 7.6
Specific questions to ask the patient: dandruff

Question	Relevance
Presence of erythema	• Dandruff is not associated with scalp redness unless the person has been scratching • Redness is characteristic of psoriasis and is common in adult seborrhoeic dermatitis
Itch	• No itch suggests psoriasis and seborrhoeic dermatitis • Itching scalp suggests dandruff
Presence of other skin lesions	• If only the scalp is involved suggests dandruff or psoriasis • Facial and trunk involvement suggests adult seborrhoeic dermatitis

commonly involved, as are the eyebrows, eyelashes and external ear. If only scalp involvement is present then the patient might complain of severe and persistent dandruff, although scalp skin will be red.

Very unlikely causes

Tinea capitis If the problem is persistent and associated with hair loss (normally as a well-circumscribed round patch of alopecia) then fungal infection of the scalp should be considered.

 TRIGGER POINTS indicative of referral: dandruff

- OTC treatment failure with a 'medicated shampoo'.
- Suspected fungal infection.

Evidence of OTC medicine efficacy

The use of a hypoallergenic shampoo on a daily basis will usually control mild symptoms. In more persistent and severe cases a 'medicated' shampoo can be used and include coal tar, selenium sulphide, zinc pyrithione and ketoconazole.

Coal tar (e.g. Polytar, T–Gel)

Virtually no published studies assessing coal tar efficacy for treating dandruff appear to have been conducted. Despite the lack of evidence, tar derivatives have been granted approval by the Food and Drug Agency in the US as an antidandruff agent and are found in many UK OTC products.

Selenium sulphide (e.g. Selsun)

Selenium is an effective antidandruff agent. Studies have shown it be significantly better than placebo and non-medicated shampoos.

Zinc pyrithione (e.g. Head and Shoulders)

Zinc pyrithione has been shown to exhibit antifungal properties and reduce cell turnover rates. It is believed that one or both of these properties confers its effectiveness in treating dandruff; however, very few trials have been published.

Ketoconazole (e.g. Nizoral dandruff shampoo)

Studies have shown it to be as effective but better tolerated as selenium sulphide. It has also been shown to act as a prophylactic agent in preventing relapse.

Practical prescribing

Prescribing information relating to medication for dandruff is summarised in the appendix.

HINTS AND TIPS

Hair discoloration: selenium and ketoconazole are reported to cause hair discoloration, albeit rarely. In addition, selenium can alter the colour of hair dyes.

Eczema/dermatitis

Dermatitis is characterised by sore, red and itching skin. In primary care, irritant contact and allergic dermatitis are most frequently encountered. Irritant contact dermatitis is caused by direct exposure to a substance that has a damaging effect to the skin, unlike allergic contact dermatitis, which is due to a sensitisation reaction.

Arriving at a differential diagnosis

143

The most likely cause of an itchy red rash seen in primary care is some form of dermatitis. Practitioners should therefore direct questions to confirm this diagnosis as other conditions can give rise to similar lesions and are listed below.

Probability	Cause
Most likely	Irritant contact dermatitis
Likely	Allergic dermatitis, occupational dermatitis, urticaria
Unlikely	Discoid eczema, plaque psoriasis
Very unlikely	Dishydrotic eczema (pompholyx), scabies, lichen planus

Clinical features of irritant contact dermatitis

Lesions will itch and appear red or brown. Itching is a prominent feature and often causes the patient to scratch, resulting in broken and weeping skin. The longer the condition persists, the more likely dryness and scaling of the skin is seen (Fig. 7.3).

Gaining an accurate diagnosis can be difficult because dermatitis rashes often look very similar and identifying specific causes is also hard. Table 7.7 lists some of the questions that should be asked to help determine the cause and if referral is needed.

Conditions to eliminate

Likely causes

Urticaria Urticarial rashes can result from many causes, most notably food allergies/food additives and medicines. The rash is itchy and red, like dermatitis, but resembles the rash seen when stung by a stinging nettle. The skin may be oedematous and blanches when pressed.

Allergic contact dermatitis Allergic contact dermatitis presents with similar symptoms to irritant dermatitis. However, milder involvement might be noticed on skin areas distant from where the allergen was in direct contact with the skin. The site of involvement often provides a major clue as to the identity of the allergen. For example, ear lobes and neck

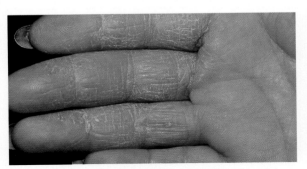

Figure 7.3 Irritant contact dermatitis. Reproduced from *Color Atlas of Dermatology* by G White, 2004, Churchill Livingstone, with permission.

Table 7.7
Specific questions to ask the patient: eczema/dermatitis

Question	Relevance
Distribution of the rash	● The distribution of rash for allergic contact dermatitis is closely associated with clothing and jewellery, e.g. watch straps, earrings, necklaces and trouser buttons/studs
Work-related exposure	● Dermatitis is often occupational. A history of when the rash occurs gives a useful indication as to the cause, e.g. a construction worker might complain of sore hands when at work but when on holiday the condition improves, only for it to worsen when he/she goes back to work
	● Exposure to chromate (found in cement and leather), rubber and hairdressing chemicals suggests an occupational cause of dermatitis

(nickel in jewellery), wrist (leather or metal watchstraps) and the feet (dyes from the tanning process of leather).

Occupational dermatitis The clinical presentation will be the same as contact irritant dermatitis. Careful enquiry about the type of work the person does and what products or equipment he or she comes into contact with should be made. In most cases if the substance can be identified a solution can usually be found, e.g. wearing gloves if dermatitis is caused by hair dyes/chemicals.

Unlikely causes

Discoid eczema This form of dermatitis usually presents in adults, who have often had a past history of atopic dermatitis. As it name implies, the lesions are circular, intensely itchy and are often distributed symmetrically on the limbs but sometimes the trunk as well.

Plaque psoriasis Plaque psoriasis classically presents with characteristic silvery-white scaly lesions of salmon-pink appearance with well-defined boundaries (Fig. 7.4). Lesions vary in size from pinpoint to covering extensive areas, and tend to exhibit symmetry affecting the elbows, knees, scalp and sacral region.

Very unlikely causes

Dishydrotic eczema (pompholyx) Pompholyx simply means 'bubble' and refers to the presence of intensely itchy vesicles or blisters on the palms of the hands and occasionally on the soles of the feet. Stress is known to precipitate the condition.

Scabies Severe pruritus on the hands and wrists is the hallmark symptom of scabies. Itching might not be localised to the hands and might worsen at night and after bathing. Blue–grey burrows up to 1 cm long might be visible but in practice they are often difficult to see.

Lichen planus The rash usually starts on the limbs and, in time, can become widespread. Lesions tend to be very itchy and exhibit flat papules. In two-thirds of patients the buccal mucosa is affected and appears as a network of white lines on its surface.

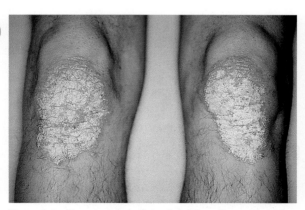

Figure 7.4 Plaque psoriasis. Reproduced from *Dermatology: An Illustrated Colour Text* by D Gawkrodger, 2002, Mosby, with permission.

Primer for differential diagnosis of dermatitis

Figure 7.5 helps to aid differentiation of dermatitis.

Figure 7.5 Primer for differential diagnosis of dermatitis.

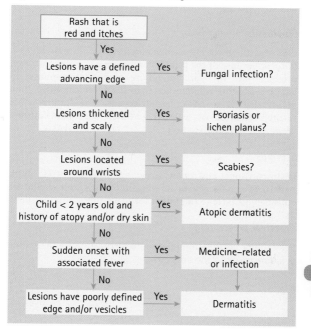

TRIGGER POINTS indicative of referral: dermatitis

- Children under 10 in need of corticosteroids.
- Lesions on the face unresponsive to emollients.
- OTC treatment failure.
- Suspected pompholyx.
- Widespread or severe dermatitis.

Evidence of OTC medicine efficacy

To varying degrees, all forms of dermatitis cause redness, drying of the skin and irritation/pruritus. Treatment should include three steps: (i) managing the itch; (ii) avoiding irritants; and (iii) maintaining skin integrity. OTC treatment of dermatitis is managed with a combination of emollients and steroid-based products.

Emollients

Choosing the most efficacious emollient for an individual is difficult because of the lack of comparative trial data between products and the variable nature of patient response. In general, patients respond better to a thicker emollient than to an elegant cosmetic brand because the former allow greater retention of water, e.g. 50% liquid paraffin/50% white soft paraffin.

Steroids

Hydrocortisone and clobetasone are available OTC. Both have proven efficacy in treating dermatitis and should be considered first line treatment for acute dermatitis.

Practical prescribing

Prescribing information relating to medication for dermatitis is summarised in the appendix.

148

HINTS AND TIPS

OTC sale of corticosteroids

There are a number of restrictions to the OTC sale of corticosteroids:

- The patient must be aged over 10 years for hydrocortisone and over 12 for clobetasone.
- Duration of treatment is limited to a maximum of 1 week.
- A maximum of 15 g can be sold at any one time.
- Corticosteroids cannot be used on facial skin, the anogenital region or broken or infected skin.

Fungal infections

Depending on the area affected, a fungal infection will manifest itself in a variety of clinical presentations. Infections are contagious and transmitted directly from one host to another.

Arriving at a differential diagnosis

Fungal infections seen in primary care include tinea pedis (athlete's foot), tinea corporis (ringworm), tinea cruris (jock itch) and tinea unguium (nail infection). Fungal infections affecting the scalp (tinea capitis), which were once common, have now declined and are very infrequently encountered. A number of other skin rashes can look superficially like fungal infections and are listed below.

Probability	Cause
Most likely	Athlete's foot
Likely	Jock itch, fungal nail infection, dermatitis
Unlikely	Psoriasis, tinea corporis
Very unlikely	Tinea capitis, tinea faciei, tinea manuum

149

Clinical features of athlete's foot

The usual site of infection is in the toe webs, especially the fourth web space (the web space next to the little toe). The skin appears white and 'soggy' (Fig. 7.6). The area is normally itchy and the feet tend to smell. The infection can spread to involve the sole, the instep of the foot or the nail. These cases are best referred.

All forms of tinea infection should be easy to recognise except isolated lesions on the body. Table 7.8 lists some of the questions that should be asked to aid diagnosis.

Conditions to eliminate

Likely causes

Tinea cruris   Tinea cruris is a fungal infection of the groin that is also known as jock itch. The rash is usually isolated

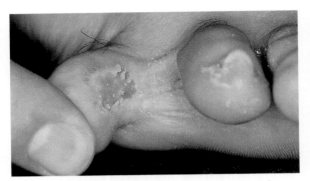

Figure 7.6 Athlete's foot. Reproduced from *Color Atlas of Dermatology* by G White, 2004, Churchill Livingstone, with permission.

Table 7.8
Specific questions to ask the patient: fungal infection

Question	Relevance
Age and sex of patient	• Athlete's foot is most prevalent in adolescents and young adults • Nail involvement usually occurs in older adults • Infection in the groin (jock itch) is much more common in men than women
Presence of itch	• Fungal infections usually itch. This usually eliminates conditions such as psoriasis, although not dermatitis/eczema
Associated symptoms	• Fungal lesions tend to be dry and scaly (except athlete's foot) and have a well-defined margin between infected and non-infected skin. Psoriasis also exhibits scaling, which tends to be thicker and more pronounced than fungal infection
Previous and family history	• No previous episodes of rash suggests tinea infection • Check for a positive family history of rash; this suggests psoriasis or ezcema

to the groin and inner thighs but can spread to the buttocks. The lesion is normally intensely itchy and reddish brown and has a well-defined edge.

Fungal nail infection   Nail involvement is relatively common if athlete's foot is persistent. The nail takes on a dull opaque and yellow appearance and over time the nail thickens, becoming more brittle and prone to crumbling (Fig. 7.7).

Dermatitis   Both fungal infections and dermatitis exhibit red itchy lesions and can therefore be difficult to distinguish from one another. Patients with dermatitis will often have a family or personal history of dermatitis and might be able to describe an event that triggered the onset of the rash.

Unlikely causes

Tinea corporis   Tinea corporis (fungal infection of the body) is defined as an infection of the major skin surfaces that do not involve the face, hands, feet, groin or scalp. The usual clinical presentation is of itchy pink or red scaly patches with a well-defined inflamed border (Fig. 7.8). The lesions often show 'central clearing' (leading edge of rash is red whilst behind is clear). Lesions can occur singly or be numerous.

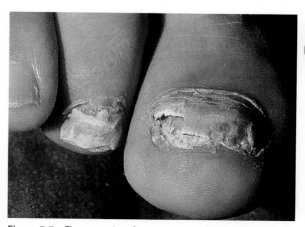

Figure 7.7   Tinea unguium (nail involvement). Reproduced from *Dermatology: An illustrated Colour Text* by D Gawkrodger, 2002, Mosby, with permission.

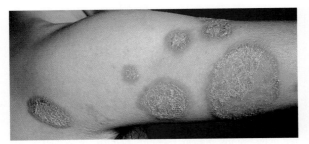

Figure 7.8   Tinea corporis. Reproduced from *Dermatology: An Illustrated Colour Text* by D Gawkrodger, 2002, Mosby, with permission.

Psoriasis   Isolated fungal body lesions can be difficult to distinguish from plaque psoriasis. However, psoriasis shows a positive family history and the lesions tend not to itch, exhibit more scaling and show symmetry.

Very unlikely causes

Tinea capitis   The first sign of infection is the appearance of a well-circumscribed round patch of alopecia that is associated with itch and scaling. Inspection of the area might reveal 'black dots' on the scalp as a result of infected hairs.

Tinea faciei   In common with tinea corporis the lesions will normally have a sharp well-defined border, show some scaling and be itchy. Facial involvement is unusual and is often initially misdiagnosed as other facial skin conditions.

Tinea manuum   Tinea manuum (fungal infection of the hand) does not look like a typical fungal infection and can therefore be misdiagnosed as eczema. The patient usually suffers from chronic diffuse scaling of one palm. Often athlete's foot will be present, as the infection is spread to the hands from the feet when the patient scratches the feet.

  TRIGGER POINTS indicative of referral: fungal infection

- Nail involvement.
- OTC treatment failure.
- Suspected facial or scalp involvement.

Evidence of OTC medicine efficacy

All tinea infections, with the exception of those involving the nails and scalp, can be treated effectively with topical OTC preparations. Although benzoic acid (Whitfield's Ointment, Toepedo) and undecenoates (e.g. Mycota) are efficacious, imidazoles (clotrimazole, miconazole, ketoconazole) and terbinafine – which have higher cure rates, quicker resolution and more cosmetically acceptable formulations – have replaced their widespread use. Trial data supporting the efficacy of tolnaftate (e.g. Mycil, Tinaderm) are limited, and tolnaftate should therefore not be routinely recommended.

Practical prescribing

Prescribing information relating to medication for fungal infections is summarised in the appendix.

HINTS AND TIPS

Length of treatment
- Miconazole: treatment should continue for 10 days after lesions cleared.
- Ketoconazole: treatment should continue for 2–3 days after lesions cleared.
- Clotrimazole: treatment should continue for 10–14 days after lesions cleared.
- Tolnaftate/undecenoates: treatment should continue for 7 days after lesions cleared.

153

Hydrocortisone–containing products (e.g. Daktacort and Canesten HC)
Hydrocortisone product licence restrictions limit treatment to 7 days. As many fungal infections will take longer than 7 days to clear, and treatment has to be typically kept up for a week or more after the lesions have cleared, to prevent reinfection, this limits the usefulness of hydrocortisone-containing products. To keep within the product licence the product would have to be discontinued after 7 days and therapy that does not contain hydrocortisone instigated.

Hair loss

Hair loss affects both men and women, although men are affected more and experience more severe hair loss. A positive family history is common and the nature and extent of hair loss will follow identical patterns as the patient's immediate parents and grandparents.

Arriving at a differential diagnosis

Diagnosis should be relatively straightforward. Androgenetic alopecia (male-pattern baldness) is the most common form of hair loss. Practitioners should therefore direct questions to confirm this diagnosis as there are a number of other conditions that cause hair loss; these are listed below.

Probability	Cause
Most likely	Male-pattern baldness
Likely	Postpartum, iron deficiency, medicine induced, stress
Unlikely	Traction alopecia, underlying medical problems, alopecia areata
Very unlikely	Tinea capitis, trichotillomania

154

Clinical features of male–pattern baldness

Men initially notice a thinning of the hair and a frontal receding hairline, which may or may not be accompanied by hair loss at the crown. Women suffer from diffuse hair loss, which is somewhat accentuated at the crown, but retain their frontal hairline. Table 7.9 lists some of the questions that should be asked to help determine if referral is needed.

Conditions to eliminate

Likely causes

Postpartum During pregnancy, hair growth increases due to increasing circulating levels of oestrogen, but after delivery of the baby oestrogen levels return to normal and the hair is shed. Patients can believe that they are experiencing

Table 7.9
Specific questions to ask the patient: hair loss

Question	Relevance
Hair loss accompanied by other symptoms	• Itch and erythema suggest fungal infection or psoriasis • Male-pattern baldness is not associated with other symptoms
Pattern of hair loss	• Frontal and crown hair loss suggests male-pattern baldness • Hair loss affecting the occipital, parietal and crown regions suggests a fungal infection • Generalised hair loss can result from stress or alopecia areata
Medical history	• A number of endocrine conditions can cause hair loss, most notably thyroid disorders
Presentation	• Unexplained hair loss can be caused by a stressful event, following surgery or after trauma • Gradual hair loss suggests male-pattern baldness • Cytotoxics (and lithium) will cause hair loss in 1–2 months

155

hair loss when in reality the hair is returning to the normal prepregnancy state. Reassurance should be given to the patient that this is a temporary and self-limiting problem.

Stress Stress is known to induce hair loss. Enquiry to ascertain lifestyle factors that might have caused recent stress and anxiety should be made.

Iron deficiency Iron deficiency is associated with female hair loss. If no other cause can be attributed to hair loss then a 2-month course of iron supplementation should result in thickening of the hair. If no response is seen, the patient should be reassessed.

Medicine-induced causes Many medicines can interfere with the hair cycle and cause transient hair loss, cytotoxic medicines being one of the most obvious examples. However, other medicines are also associated with hair loss:

- anticoagulants (up to 50% of patients)
- lithium carbonate (up to 10% of patients)
- interferons (20–30% of patients)
- oral contraceptives (2–3 months after discontinuation of the product)
- retinoids (up to 20% of patients).

Unlikely causes

Traction alopecia Most commonly seen in women, traction alopecia refers to hair loss due to excess and sustained tension on the hair, usually as a result of styling hair with rollers or a particular type of hairstyle.

Underlying endocrine disorder Diabetes mellitus, hypopituitarism and hypothyroidism can result in poor hair growth. In hypothyroidism the hair is thin and brittle and the patient might be lethargic and have a history of recent weight gain.

Alopecia areata Unlike androgenetic alopecia, the hair loss is sudden and affects mainly children and adolescents. It can involve only small patches of hair loss or the whole scalp might be affected. The condition is usually self-limiting and regrowth of hair is often observed, although repeated episodes are not unusual.

156

Very unlikely causes

Fungal scalp infection (tinea capitis) The first sign of infection is the appearance of a well-circumscribed round patch of alopecia that is associated with itch and scaling. Inspection of the area may reveal 'black dots' on the scalp as a result of infected hairs.

Trichotillomania This refers to patients who have an impulsive desire to twist and pull scalp hair. The patient usually has some form of psychiatric illness and it would be very unusual for such patients not to already be known to the GP/psychiatric team.

TRIGGER POINTS indicative of referral: hair loss

- Fungal infection of the scalp.
- Patients under 18 years old.
- Possible endocrine cause.
- Suspected iron deficiency for blood test.
- Trichotillomania.

Evidence of OTC medicine efficacy

Currently, minoxidil is the only product OTC for male-pattern baldness. It is available as either a 2% or 5% solution.

A number of clinical trials have investigated the efficacy and safety of minoxidil. Trial results are not totally convincing. Minoxidil is superior to placebo (although placebo does invoke a large initial response) but longitudinal studies show that less than half of patients treated experience moderate to marked hair growth, and by 30 months hair counts have decreased (albeit still above baseline) and the bald area increases back in size to its initial diameter. In women, the situation is not too dissimilar, although the 5% solution offers no advantage over the 2% solution. In summary, minoxidil will promote hair growth in approximately 50% of minimally balding young men but over time the effect tails off. After 30 months the effect is still greater than baseline but, on the whole, will not achieve cosmetically acceptable hair growth.

Practical prescribing

Prescribing information relating to minoxidil is summarised in the appendix.

HINTS AND TIPS

- Minoxidil absorption: systemic circulation may occur and can result in chest pain, rapid heartbeat, faintness or dizziness.

Psoriasis

Psoriasis is a chronic relapsing inflammatory disorder that affects up to 2% of the UK population. It most commonly occurs in young adults and there is often a family history. It is characterised by a variety of morphological lesions that present in a number of forms.

Arriving at a differential diagnosis

The most common forms of psoriasis seen in primary care are plaque and scalp psoriasis. Practitioners should therefore direct questions to establish whether these are the cause as other rashes can appear similar to psoriasis, and are listed below.

Probability	Cause
Most likely	Plaque psoriasis, scalp psoriasis
Likely	Seborrhoeic dermatitis, tinea infections (except scalp)
Unlikely	Pustular, guttate and flexural psoriasis, pityriasis rosea, medication
Very unlikely	Erythrodermic psoriasis, lichen planus, tinea capitis

158

Clinical features of plaque and scalp psoriasis

Plaque psoriasis classically presents with characteristic silvery-white scaly lesions of salmon-pink appearance with well-defined boundaries (see Fig. 7.4). Lesions exhibit symmetry, affecting elbows, knees and sacral areas, and vary in size from pinpoint to covering extensive areas. Scalp psoriasis can be mild, exhibiting slight redness of the scalp, through to severe cases with marked inflammation and thick scaling. The redness often extends beyond the hair margin and is commonly seen behind the ears. Table 7.10 lists some of the questions that should be asked to determine diagnosis or if referral is needed.

Table 7.10
Specific questions to ask the patient: psoriasis

Question	Relevance
Age	<ul><li>Rash that develops in early adulthood suggests psoriasis</li><li>Lichen planus usually affects people aged 30–60 years</li><li>Guttate psoriasis occurs in adolescents</li></ul>
Distribution of rash	<ul><li>Lesions showing symmetry suggest psoriasis</li><li>Lesions seen on the inside of the wrists suggests lichen planus</li><li>Lesions on the thighs and trunk suggests pityriasis rosea</li></ul>
Other symptoms	<ul><li>Slight itch suggests psoriasis</li><li>Prominent/intense itching suggests dermatitis or fungal infection</li><li>Nail pitting and separation of the nail plate from the nail bed suggests psoriasis (only patients with long-standing psoriasis)</li></ul>
Look of rash	<ul><li>Scaling lesions are a prominent feature in psoriasis</li><li>Scaling also occurs in pityriasis rosea and adult seborrhoeic dermatitis but not to the same extent as in psoriasis</li></ul>
Previous history of lesions	<ul><li>If patients have had similar lesions in the past this suggests psoriasis</li><li>No previous history suggests conditions such as fungal infection and pityriasis rosea</li></ul>

159

Conditions to eliminate

Likely causes

Seborrhoeic dermatitis Mild scalp psoriasis can be very difficult to distinguish from seborrhoeic dermatitis. However, in practice this is rarely a problem because treatment for both conditions is often the same.

Tinea corporis The usual clinical presentation is of itchy pink or red scaly patches with a well-defined inflamed border (see Fig. 7.8). The lesions often show 'central clearing' (leading edge of rash is red, behind is clear). Lesions can occur singly or be numerous.

Unlikely causes

Pustular psoriasis In this form of psoriasis sterile pustules are an obvious clinical feature. The pustules tend to be located on the advancing edge of the lesions and typically occur on the palms of the hands and soles of the feet.

Flexural psoriasis Flexural psoriasis refers to classic lesions that affect the scalp but also lesions in the body folds, especially the groins and axillae, which are smooth with minimal scaling.

Guttate psoriasis Guttate psoriasis is characterised by crops of scattered small lesions covered with light flaky scales that often affect the trunk and proximal part of the limbs. This form of psoriasis usually occurs in adolescents and often follows a streptococcal throat infection.

Pityriasis rosea The condition is characterised by erythematous scaling mainly on the trunk, but also on the thighs and upper arms. A 'target' disc lesion, often misdiagnosed as a fungal infection, is followed 1 week later by an extensive rash. It most commonly affects young adults. The condition usually remits spontaneously after 4–8 weeks.

Medication that can trigger or aggravate psoriasis A number of medicines can cause rashes that look like psoriasis or aggravate existing psoriasis. These include lithium, betablockers, chloroquine, terbinafine and steroid withdrawal.

Very unlikely causes

Erythrodermic psoriasis Erythrodermic psoriasis presents as an extensive erythema and shows very few classic lesions; it is therefore difficult to diagnosis. The condition is serious and even life-threatening. Systemic symptoms can be severe and include fever, joint pain and diarrhoea.

Lichen planus The lesions are similar in appearance to plaque psoriasis but are usually itchy and normally located on the inner surfaces of the wrists and shins. Additionally, oral mucous membranes are normally affected with white, slightly raised lesions that look a little like a spider's web.

Tinea capitis Tinea capitis (fungal infection of the scalp) is an uncommon infection but if the patient has scaling skin, broken hairs and a patch of alopecia then a tinea infection should be considered.

Primer for differential diagnosis of plaque psoriasis

Figure 7.9 aids in the differentiation of plaque psoriasis.

> **TRIGGER POINTS indicative of referral: psoriasis**
>
> - Lesions that are extensive, follow recent infection or cause moderate to severe itching.
> - Patients with no family history or past personal history of psoriasis.
> - Pustular psoriatic lesions.

Figure 7.9 Primer for differential diagnosis of plaque psoriasis.

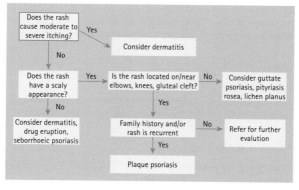

Evidence of OTC medicine efficacy

OTC treatment should be limited to mild to moderate plaque psoriasis and scalp psoriasis. Treatment consists of emollients, keratolytics, coal tar or dithranol. There is limited published literature supporting efficacy of topical treatment; however, other topical products which are more effective (e.g. calcipotriol) can be obtained on prescription.

Emollients

No published literature appears to have addressed emollient efficacy or whether one emollient is superior to another. Despite this, subjective evidence over a long period of time has shown that emollients are useful for mild psoriasis and are an important aspect of treatment.

Keratolytics

Keratolytics have been used to aid clearing scale and are often used for scalp psoriasis, in which very thick scaling can occur. Although there appears to be no published evidence for their efficacy, clinical practice suggests that they have a role to play.

Coal tar

A number of clinical studies have confirmed the beneficial effect coal tar has on psoriasis although a major drawback in assessing the effectiveness of coal tar is the lack of comparison trials between different products. It is therefore difficult to know if any product is superior to another.

Dithranol

Dithranol has proven efficacy. Current practice dictates starting on the lowest possible concentration and gradually increasing the concentration until improvement is noticed.

Practical prescribing

Prescribing information relating to medication for psoriasis is summarised in the appendix.

HINTS AND TIPS

- Use of emollients: all emollients should be regularly and liberally applied with no upper limit on how often they can be used.
- Application of dithranol: short contact therapy is often advocated for dithranol because prolonged exposure can lead to irritation and burning skin. This involves using the lowest strength available (0.1%) for 30 minutes, which is then washed off. Gradually the concentration of dithranol is increased to 1%. If psoriasis fails to respond with 1% treatment then referral to the GP is needed for higher strength treatment.

Seborrhoeic dermatitis

There are two distinct types of seborrhoeic dermatitis, the more common infantile form (known as cradle cap) and an adult form. Cradle cap usually starts before the age of 6 months and is usually self-limiting; the adult form tends to be chronic and persistent.

Arriving at a differential diagnosis

The most likely scalp condition encountered in primary care in infants is cradle cap. The adult form also affects the scalp but other areas of the skin are involved. A small number of conditions that can present with similar symptoms are listed below.

163

Probability	Cause
Most likely	Seborrhoeic dermatitis
Likely	Atopic dermatitis (in infants)
Unlikely	Psoriasis
Very unlikely	Pityriasis versicolor

Clinical features of seborrhoeic dermatitis

Cradle cap appears as large, yellow scales and crusts on the scalp but in severe cases the face and napkin area are also involved. The adult form is characterised by a red, mildly itchy, scaly rash that typically affects the central part of the face, scalp, eyebrows, eyelids, nasolabial folds and mid-chest.

Arriving at a diagnosis of cradle cap should not be too difficult but the adult form might be more problematic. Table 7.11 lists some of the questions that should be asked to help determine if referral is needed.

Conditions to eliminate

Likely causes

Atopic dermatitis A typical presentation is an irritable, scratching child with dermatitis of varying severity. In infants, atopic dermatitis usually presents as itchy lesions on the scalp, face and trunk (Fig. 7.10). Most patients will have a positive family history of the atopic triad of dermatitis, asthma or hay fever.

Unlikely causes

Psoriasis Adults who suffer from scalp psoriasis can be confused with patients with severe and persistent dandruff caused by seborrhoeic dermatitis. However, facial involvement is generally also present in seborrhoeic dermatitis unlike psoriasis.

Very unlikely causes

Pityriasis versicolor This condition usually develops after exposure to the sun. It can be mistaken for adult seborrhoeic dermatitis as the lesions exhibit fine superficial scale and are located on the trunk. However, the rash does not itch and the face is usually spared.

❗ TRIGGER POINTS indicative of referral: seborrhoeic dermatitis

- Treatment failure with OTC medicines.
- Lesions that appear after exposure to sunlight.

Table 7.11
Specific questions to ask the patient: seborrhoeic dermatitis

Question	Relevance
Age	• From birth onwards suggests cradle cap • Older infants (> 6 months) suggests atopic dermatitis
Itching	• Cradle cap does not itch. This is a useful differentiating feature between atopic and seborrhoeic dermatitis
Location	• Face and mid-chest involvement in an adult suggests seborrhoeic dermatitis • Scalp and napkin involvement suggests cradle cap • Knees and elbows in children suggests atopic dermatitis • Mainly on the body suggests pityriasis versicolor
Family history	• No family history suggests cradle cap • Family history suggests psoriasis or atopic dermatitis
Other symptoms	• Associated ear/eye problems suggests adult seborrhoeic dermatitis • A well and happy child suggests seborrhoeic dermatitis • A child who is fractious and miserable suggests atopic dermatitis • Scalp involvement shows yellow/greasy scale in cradle cap • Silvery scales suggest psoriasis
Physical signs	• Lumps in the hair suggest psoriasis • A smooth scalp suggests cradle cap

165

Evidence of OTC medicine efficacy

OTC treatment for cradle cap comprises emollients and the use of a hypoallergenic shampoo on a daily basis and will usually control mild symptoms. In more persistent and severe cases a 'medicated' shampoo can be used; these contain coal

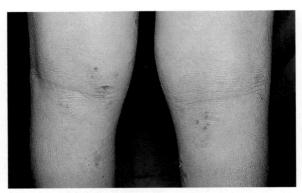

Figure 7.10 Atopic dermatitis in the popliteal fossa.
Reproduced from *Dermatology: An Illustrated Colour Text* by
D Gawkrodger, 2002, Mosby, with permission.

tar, selenium sulphide, zinc pyrithione and ketoconazole.
The adult form responds well to topical steroids but recurrence is common.

Practical prescribing

Prescribing information relating to medication for seborrhoeic dermatitis is summarised in the appendix.

Scabies

Scabies can affect anyone but is more frequently seen in the
elderly. It is caused by the mite *Sarcoptes scabiei* and is
transmitted by direct physical contact. The incidence of
scabies in the UK is low but epidemics can occur on a
cyclical basis every 7–15 years.

Arriving at a differential diagnosis

Marked itching involving the hands is most likely to be
scabies. Practitioners should direct questions to establish
whether this is the cause, as confusion can arise from mis-
taking scabies for dermatitis or dermatitis herpetiformis.

Probability	Cause
Most likely	Scabies
Likely	Dermatitis
Unlikely	Dermatitis herpetiformis

Clinical features of scabies

Severe pruritus on the hands and wrists is the hallmark symptom of scabies. Itching might not be localised to the hands and might worsen at night and after bathing. In men, the penile and scrotal skin, and in women the skin beneath the breasts and nipples, can also be affected. Blue–grey burrows up to 1 cm long might be visible but in practice are difficult to see.

The diagnosis of scabies is confirmed by extraction of the mite from its burrow, but in primary care this is rarely performed. Diagnosis is made on clinical appearance, patient history and symptoms reported by close family. Table 7.12 lists questions that should be asked to help determine the best course of action.

Table 7.12
Specific questions to ask the patient: scabies

Question	Relevance
Location of rash	• If the finger webs, the sides of the fingers and the wrists are involved this suggests scabies • Hand involvement is rare in dermatitis herpetiformis
History of presenting complaint	• A prior history of lesions suggests contact dermatitis • Certain people, e.g. care workers looking after institutionalised people, are at more risk of getting scabies

Conditions to eliminate

Likely causes

Dermatitis The condition presents as an area of inflamed, itchy skin with either papules or vesicles being present. An allergen might be identified as to the cause of the rash (perfume, watch straps, etc.) and there might be milder involvement on areas away from the hands.

Unlikely causes

Dermatitis herpetiformis Dermatitis herpetiformis is a chronic condition that affects mainly young adults and is characterised by intense itchy clusters of papules and vesicles that exhibit a symmetrical distribution. It commonly involves the elbows, knees and sacral region.

TRIGGER POINTS indicative of referral: scabies

- Severe and extensive symptoms.
- Suspected dermatitis herpetiformis.

Evidence of OTC medicine efficacy

The efficacy and safety of scabicidal agents is difficult to determine. Benzyl benzoate, crotamiton, permethrin and malathion have all been used. The current edition of the *BNF* (edition 47) advocates the use of permethrin and malathion.

A Cochrane review (Walker et al, *Cochrane Review* issue 2, 1999) found permethrin to have cure rates of approximately 90%. This review also compared permethrin against other scabicidal agents and concluded that it was superior to crotamiton and equally effective as gamma-benzene hexachloride (the latter was withdrawn from the UK market in 1995 because of concern about possible adverse effects). The efficacy of malathion is questionable as no randomised controlled trials appear to have been conducted but case reports suggest malathion is effective with cure rates > 80%. In uncontrolled trials benzyl benzoate has shown to provide cure rates of approximately 50%. Unfortunately, up to 25% of patients experience side-effects such as burning, irritation and itching on application.

Practical prescribing

Prescribing information relating to medication for scabies is summarised in the appendix.

> **HINTS AND TIPS**
>
> **Application of products**
> - In children up to 2 years of age: apply to whole body except the face.
> - In people > 2 years of age: apply to the whole body, including the face.
> - Permethrin: wash off after 8–12 hours.
> - Malathion: wash off after 24 hours.

Warts and verrucas

Warts and verrucas are benign, self-limiting growths of the skin caused by the human papillomavirus (HPV). They have a peak incidence in children and are uncommon in the elderly. They should not be picked, bitten or scratched as this can lead to multiple lesions.

Arriving at a differential diagnosis

Warts and verrucas are not difficult to diagnose yet a number of similar conditions seen in primary care superficially look like warts and verrucas and are listed below.

Probability	Cause
Most likely	Common wart/verruca
Likely	Plane wart, molluscum contagiosum, corns
Unlikely	Seborrhoeic wart, mosaic wart
Very unlikely	Basal cell carcinoma

Clinical features of warts and verrucas

Warts occur on the hands and knees either singly or in crops. When examined, the wart appears as a raised, hyperkeratotic papule with thrombosed, black vessels visible as black dots within it (Fig. 7.11). Verrucas grow inwards rather than outwards because of the constant pressure exerted by the foot on the verruca. Inspection of the lesion will normally reveal tiny black dots on the surface (Fig. 7.12). Pressure on nerves can cause pain when walking.

Table 7.13 lists some of the questions that should be asked to help determine the diagnosis. (It is worth noting that HPV infections involving the anogenital area should be dealt with by a GP.)

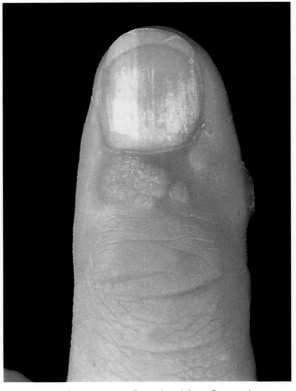

Figure 7.11   Common wart. Reproduced from *Dermatology Colour Guide* by J Wilkinson and S Shaw, 1998, Churchill Livingstone, with permission.

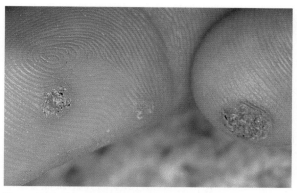

Figure 7.12 Verruca. Reproduced from *Dermatology: An Illustrated Colour Text* by D Gawkrodger, 2002, Mosby, with permission.

Conditions to eliminate

Likely causes

Plane warts (flat warts or verruca plana) These most frequently occur on the face and the back of the hands. They are small in size (1–5 mm in diameter), slightly raised and can take on the skin colour of the patient (Fig. 7.13).

Molluscum contagiosum Molluscum contagiosum primarily affects children under 5 years old. Patients present with multiple lesions, usually on the face and neck, although the trunk can also be involved (Fig. 7.14). The lesions resemble common warts, but each raised papule tends to be smooth and have a central dimple; the latter is a useful diagnostic point. The condition is self-limiting and will resolve without medical intervention.

Corns Hard corns and plantar warts can be confused. Corns are generally located on the tops of the toes (an unusual place for verrucas) and appear as a painful, raised, yellow ring of inflammatory skin with a central core of hard grey skin.

Unlikely causes

Seborrhoeic wart (basal cell papilloma) Basal cell papillomas are benign growths that usually affect the elderly. They

Table 7.13
**Specific questions to ask the patient:
warts and verrucas**

Question	Relevance
Age of patient	• A raised lesion in children under 10 suggests a wart
	• The likelihood that nodular lesions are caused by seborrhoeic warts or carcinoma increases with increasing age
Location	• Warts are common on the hands and knees; verrucas are usually found on the weight-bearing parts of the sole
	• Warts can occur on the face but should be referred as OTC treatment can cause scarring
	• In the elderly, warts on the face can suggest cancer: **refer**
	• Lesions on the face and body suggests molluscum contagiosum
Associated symptoms	• Itching and bleeding are not associated with warts and verrucas and must be viewed with suspicion, especially in older patients
	• Pain on walking suggests a verruca
Colour/appearance	• Typically warts have a 'cauliflower' appearance and are raised and pale
	• Warts with a reddish hue or that change colour should be referred
	• Lesions that are raised, smooth and have a central 'dimple' suggest molluscum contagiosum

appear as raised often multiple brown lesions and have a superficial 'stuck on' appearance (Fig. 7.15).

Mosaic warts Occasionally, a number of closely located verrucas can coalesce to form a large single plaque called a mosaic wart. Referral is often required.

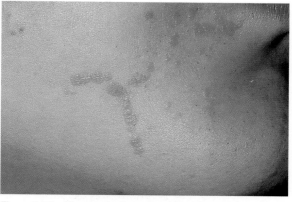

Figure 7.13 Plane warts. Reproduced from *Dermatology: An Illustrated Colour Text* by D Gawkrodger, 2002, Mosby, with permission.

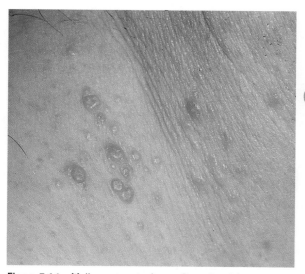

Figure 7.14 Molluscum contagiosum. Reproduced from *Dermatology: An Illustrated Colour Text* by D Gawkrodger, 2002, Mosby, with permission.

173

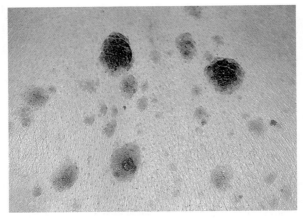

Figure 7.15 Seborrhoeic wart. Reproduced from *Dermatology: An Illustrated Colour Text* by D Gawkrodger, 2002, Mosby, with permission.

Very unlikely causes

Basal cell carcinoma   Skin cancers typically occur in older age groups. Often there will be a history of prolonged skin exposure. Any wart-like lesion that is itchy, has an irregular outline, is prone to bleeding and exhibits colour change should be referred to eliminate serious pathology.

174

Evidence of OTC medicine efficacy

The most commonly used agent found in OTC treatments is salicylic acid, both alone and in combination. Salicylic acid

> TRIGGER POINTS indicative of referral: warts and verrucas
>
> - Anogenital warts.
> - Diabetic patients.
> - Lesions on the face.
> - Multiple and widespread warts.
> - Patients aged over 50 presenting with a first time wart.
> - Warts that itch or bleed without provocation.
> - Warts that have grown and/or changed colour.

has been shown to heal 60–80% of lesions after 12 weeks, although there appear to be no trials comparing cure rates with different concentrations. In addition, salicylic acid/lactic acid combinations appear to show no greater efficacy than salicylic acid alone. There is some evidence to show that common warts are more responsive to keratolytic therapy than plantar warts, and healing might be helped by soaking the wart or verruca prior to application and/or occlusion of the site to aid penetration.

Other products OTC include formaldehyde, glutaraldehyde, podophyllum resin and silver nitrate pencils. Information regarding their effectiveness stems from either small-scale or poorly designed studies and their use should therefore be relegated to second-line choices. However, it should be noted that cure rates reported with these agents, except silver nitrate, were equal to if not better than those reported with salicylic acid.

Practical prescribing

Prescribing information relating to medication for warts and verrucas is summarised in the appendix.

HINTS AND TIPS

Symptom resolution
● Over half of all common warts and verrucas will resolve spontaneously after 2 years, therefore treatment is not necessarily needed.

Associated problems with application
● Glutaraldehyde can stain the outer layer of the skin brown.
● Wartner (containing propane and dimethylether) has recently been introduced in to the UK. It has the same action as liquid nitrogen in that it 'freezes' the wart. Obvious care is needed when applying the product to ensure that healthy skin is not frozen and the product is not left in contact with the wart for too long (maximum 20 seconds). Assessment of patient understanding and dexterity would be prudent before recommendation/purchase. If doubts exist then referral to the GP for cryotherapy should be considered.

Chapter 8

Musculoskeletal conditions

The musculoskeletal system comprises tissues that are hard (bone and cartilage) and soft (muscles, tendons, ligaments). At the point of contact between two or more bones a joint is formed. This system of bones and joints maximises movement while maintaining stability.

Acute low back pain

Acute low back pain is self-limiting, with more than 90% of cases resolving within 6 weeks, although relapse is common. Patients aged 20–50 years are most likely to suffer and certain groups, e.g. industrial workers and people who play sports, are more prone to back pain.

Arriving at a differential diagnosis

The most likely cause of back pain seen in primary care for all ages is related to physical activity. Practitioners should therefore direct questions to confirm this diagnosis as other conditions cause back pain and are listed below.

Probability	Cause
Most likely	Simple back pain associated with physical activity
Likely	Nerve root compression (e.g. sciatica), pregnancy, osteoarthritis
Unlikely	Osteomyelitis, compression fractures
Very unlikely	Malignancy

Clinical features of acute low back pain

Patients present with symptoms that came on quickly; they will have reduced mobility and pain described as aching or stiffness. Depending on the cause, pain might be localised, e.g. lumbosacral strains following physical activity, or more diffuse, e.g. from postural backache after sitting incorrectly for a prolonged period.

Although more than 95% of cases will be simple back pain, it is important to rule out more sinister causes so that appropriate referrals can be made. Table 8.1 lists some of the questions that should be asked to aid differential diagnosis.

Conditions to eliminate

Likely causes

Sciatica   Low back pain is accompanied by pain that radiates to the upper leg. If the disc presses on the nerve then pain can shoot down the leg (like an electric shock) reaching as far as the foot. Coughing, sneezing or straining at stool often aggravates pain.

Unlikely causes

Osteomyelitis   Back pain associated with fever that worsens with activity is suggestive of infection. The patient should be referred to the GP for blood tests.

Compression fractures   These can occur with minimal trauma, especially in the elderly. Pain should be acute in onset and is in either the lower back or pelvic region.

Very unlikely causes

178

Malignancy   A history of significant weight loss and the presence of anaemia, general malaise, night pain and symptoms that do not improve suggest malignancy, especially if the person is aged over 50 years.

Chronic causes of low back pain

It is worth remembering that many patients suffer from chronic back pain (> 3 months' duration) and might ask for advice. Degenerative joint disease (e.g. osteoarthritis) in older patients is common. Onset of deep aching pain is gradual and is characterised by early-morning stiffness.

Table 8.1
Specific questions to ask the patient: back pain

Question	Relevance
Age	The most likely diagnosis will vary with age: ● < 15 years: specific/serious causes found in up to 50% of patients: **refer** ● 15–30 years: prolapsed disc, trauma, fractures and pregnancy ● 30–50 years: degenerative joint disease (osteoarthritis), prolapsed disc and malignancy ● > 50 years: osteoporosis, malignancy and metabolic bone disorders (Paget's disease)
Location	● Pain that radiates into the buttocks, thighs and legs suggests nerve root compression: **refer**
Onset	● Acute and sudden in onset suggests muscle strain in the lumbosacral region ● Acute low back pain in the elderly should be referred as even slight trauma can result in compression fractures ● Low back pain that is insidious in onset should be viewed with caution as it may suggest malignancy: **refer**
Restriction of movement	● Difficulty in sitting down suggests disc herniation: **refer** ● Pain exacerbated by physical activity and relieved by rest suggests a mechanical cause, e.g. muscle strain ● Pain that is worse when resting and disturbs sleep suggests a systemic cause: **refer**
Predisposing factors	● Bad posture while seated and poor lifting technique when performing day-to-day tasks can precipitate back pain

179

> **!** TRIGGER POINTS indicative of referral: low back pain

- Associated fever.
- Back pain from structures above the lumbar region.
- Failure to improve 10–14 days after onset.
- Numbness.
- Patients under 20 and over 60.
- Persistent and progressively worsening pain.
- Referred pain into the lower leg.
- Suspected fracture.

Evidence of OTC efficacy

Conservative treatment

A number of systematic reviews have shown bed rest to be counterproductive. Patients might benefit from short-term rest, lasting no longer than 2 days, after which they should be encouraged to exercise.

Analgesics

All systemic analgesics when prescribed as monotherapy (paracetamol, aspirin, ibuprofen) have proven efficacy in pain relief at standard doses. However, the use of non-steroidal anti-inflammatory drugs for 7–10 days is widely advocated. Compound analgesics (paracetamol/codeine, aspirin/codeine or paracetamol/dihydrocodeine) contain low doses of opiates, and a number of papers have concluded that OTC doses of opiates are too low to produce statistically significant reductions in pain compared with single agents.

Caffeine is included in a number of proprietary products, but claims that caffeine enhances analgesic efficacy have not been substantiated.

Topical therapy

Non-steroidal anti-inflammatory drugs
Prior to 1998, publications such as *MeReC* and *The Drug and Therapeutics Bulletin* stated that trial data on topical non-steroidal anti-inflammatory drugs (NSAIDs) were questionable. However, a systematic review (Moore et al, *BMJ* 1998;

316: 333–338) involving > 10 000 patients concluded that topical non-steroidal anti-inflammatory drugs were effective and had a lower incidence of side-effects than the same drugs taken orally.

Rubefacients

There is no evidence to support their effect (except capsaicin), and rubefacients should not be routinely recommended as first-line treatment. Capsaicin (as two POM products, Axsain and Zacin) has been granted product licences for certain conditions associated with pain. Although these formulations are not available OTC, a number of OTC products do contain capsaicin (e.g. Balmosa and Ralgex) at concentrations equivalent or higher than those found in the POM products. Although no evidence exists for these products in relieving pain, it would seem reasonable to suppose that they may show similar effects. Trials are therefore needed to determine if OTC products are effective.

Summary

Based on evidence, patients with acute low back pain should be encouraged to exercise and be given a short course of a systemic non-steroidal anti-inflammatory drug unless contraindicated. Topical non-steroidal anti-inflammatory drugs could also be recommended for those patients in whom side-effects need to be minimised.

HINTS AND TIPS

- Asthmatics: in a small minority of asthmatic patients aspirin can precipitate shortness of breath, therefore any asthmatic who has previously had a hypersensitivity reaction to aspirin should avoid both aspirin and ibuprofen.
- Children and aspirin: aspirin-taking in children has been linked to Reye's syndrome, a rare syndrome in which encephalopathy can occur, which, if not diagnosed early, can lead to death. No child under 16 years should be given aspirin.
- Topical products: gentle massage of the area on application might be beneficial in dissipating swelling and help reduce pain, therefore products with no evidence base might still prove useful.

Practical prescribing

Prescribing information relating to medication for back pain is summarised in the appendix and proprietary analgesic products are listed in Table 8.2.

Activity/sports-related soft tissue injuries

Sprains (overstretching or twisting of ligaments) and strains (tearing of muscle fibres) are most likely to be seen in primary care.

Arriving at a differential diagnosis

Most commonly affected sites of injury are the ankles and knees, with fewer cases affecting the shoulders or elbows. The most commonly encountered problems seen in primary care are listed below.

	Shoulder	*Elbow*	*Knee*	*Ankle*
Most likely	Frozen shoulder	Epicondylitis	Ligament damage	Ankle sprains
Likely	Rotator cuff syndrome	Bursitis	Runner's knee	Achilles tendon injuries
Unlikely	Repetitive strain injury	Stress fractures	Stress fractures	Plantar fasciitis, stress fractures, gout

Clinical features of soft tissue injury

In general, patients will present with pain, swelling and bruising. The extent of symptoms will be determined by the severity of the injury. Knowing the site of the injury will, in part, dictate the type of questions asked. Table 8.3 outlines some of the questions that should be asked to aid diagnosis.

Most likely causes

Frozen shoulder This term is used to describe when the shoulder has marked restriction in all the major ranges of motion. It often occurs without warning or explanation.

Table 8.2
Proprietary analgesics available OTC

Product	Aspirin	Paracetamol	Ibuprofen	Codeine	Other	Children
Advil			200 mg			>12 years
Alka-Seltzer XS	267 mg	133 mg			Caffeine 40 mg	>16 years
Alka-Xs Go	300 mg	200 mg			Caffeine 45 mg	>16 years
Anadin Extra tabs/sol tabs	300 mg	200 mg			Caffeine 45 mg	>16 years
Anadin Ibuprofen			200 mg			>12 years
Anadin Paracetamol		500 mg				>6 years
Anadin	325 mg				Caffeine 15 mg	>16 years
Anadin Ultra			200 mg			>12 years
Askit Powders	530 mg				Aloxiprin 140 mg Caffeine 110 mg	>16 years

table continues

183

Table 8.2 continued

Product	Aspirin	Paracetamol	Ibuprofen	Codeine	Other	Children
Aspro Clear	300 mg					>16 years
Calpol products		120 or 250 mg				>3 months
Codis 500	500 mg			8 mg		>16 years
Cuprofen			200 mg			>12 years
Cuprofen maximum			400 mg			>12 years
Disprin and Disprin Direct	300 mg					>16 years
Disprin Extra	300 mg	200 mg				>16 years
Disprol products		120 mg				>3 months
Hedex		500 mg				>6 years
Hedex Extra		500 mg			Caffeine 65 mg	>12 years
Hedex Ibuprofen			200 mg			>12 years
Medinol products		120 or 250 mg				>3 months

184

Product						Age
Nurofen tabs, meltabs, liquid caps and caplets			200 mg			>12 years
Nurofen Long Lasting			300 mg			>12 years
Nurofen Plus			200 mg		12.8 mg	>12 years
Nurse Sykes Powders	165 mg	120 mg		Caffeine 65 mg		>16 years
Panadol tabs and Actifast tabs	500 mg					>12 years
Panadol Extra tabs and sol. tabs	500 mg			Caffeine 65 mg		>12 years
Panadol Night	500 mg			Diphenhydramine 25 mg		>12 years
Panadol Ultra	500 mg				12.8 mg	>12 years
Paracodol tabs and sol. tabs	500 mg				8 mg	>12 years
Paramol		521 mg		Dihydrocodeine 7.46 mg		>12 years
Phensic			325 mg	Caffeine 22 mg		>16 years

table continues

Table 8.2 continued

Product	Aspirin	Paracetamol	Ibuprofen	Codeine	Other	Children
Propain		400 mg			Caffeine 50 mg Diphenhydramine 5 mg	>16 years
Solpadeine tabs/caps/sol. tabs		500 mg		8 mg	Caffeine 30 mg	>12 years
Solpadeine Max		500 mg		12.8 mg		>12 years
Solpaflex			200 mg	12.8 mg		>12 years
Syndol		450 mg		10 mg	Caffeine 30 mg Doxylamine 5 mg	>12 years
Veganin		500 mg		8 mg	Caffeine 30 mg	>12 years

Table 8.3
Specific questions to ask the patient: soft tissue injuries

Question	Relevance
Who is the patient	• Sports-related injuries usually affect the knees and ankles • Elderly people often sustain injuries through falls
Timing	• When did it happen and when did the patient present? The closer these two events are, the more serious the injury
Presenting symptoms	• Marked swelling, bruising and pain that occurs straight after injury suggests more serious injury: **refer**
Nature of injury	• The greater the force of impact, the greater the chance of fracture • Sudden onset, associated with a single traumatic event suggests tendon/ligament damage
Range of motion	• A marked reduction in normal range of motion of the affected joint suggests major trauma: **refer**
Nature of pain	• Referred pain suggests nerve root compression, e.g. a shoulder injury in which pain is also felt in the hand: **refer**
Age of patient	• Insidious and progressive pain suggests some form of degenerative disease: **refer** • Children and the elderly are more prone to fractures and are probably best referred

Non-steroidal anti-inflammatory drugs could be offered, but if symptoms fail to respond after 5 days' treatment referral for alternative treatment and physiotherapy should be considered.

Ankle sprains The ankle acts as a hinge joint, permitting up and down motion. Three sets of ligaments provide stability to the joint: the deltoid, lateral collateral and syndesmosis. The majority of ankle sprains involve the lateral ligamentous structures due to inversion of the joint (twisted ankles). Most patients will walk with a limp because the ankle cannot support their full weight.

Knee ligament damage Find out from the patient how the injury occurred. If the injury occurred when twisting, this implies damage to medial meniscus. This is less serious than damage to the anterior cruciate ligament, which usually occurs when the person receives a blow to the back of the knee.

Epicondylitis Two main presentations of epicondylitis are seen: tennis elbow (lateral epicondylitis) and golfer's elbow (medial epicondylitis). Tennis elbow is characterised by pain felt over the outer aspect of the elbow joint; the pain may spread up the upper arm. The patient will have a history of gradually increasing pain and tenderness. In comparison, pain of golfer's elbow is noticed on the inner side of the elbow and can radiate down the forearm. Both names are misleading as people other than tennis and golf players can suffer from the problems, which are usually related to a repetitive activity.

Conditions to eliminate

Likely causes

Rotator cuff syndrome The rotator cuff refers to the combined tendons of the scapula muscles that hold the head of the humerus in place. Rubbing these tendons causes pain. It is most often seen in patients over the age of 40 and is associated with repetitive overhead activity. Pain tends to worsen at night and may disturb sleep. Reaching behind the back also tends to worsen pain.

Achilles tendon injuries Injuries to the structures associated with the Achilles tendon is usually seen in runners (when increasing their mileage or running over hilly terrain) or athletes involved in jumping sports. Pain is felt behind and above the heel, and progressively worsens the longer the injury lasts.

Runner's knee (chondromalacia)   Most commonly noted in recreational joggers who are increasing mileage, e.g. someone training to run the marathon. It develops insidiously, with pain being the predominant symptom. Pain can be aggravated by prolonged periods of sitting down in the same position or climbing stairs. Treatment depends on the severity of pain: non-steroidal anti-inflammatory drugs can be used if the pain is mild but total rest and stopping running is required if the pain is severe.

Bursitis of the elbow (student's elbow)   Bursae can become inflamed leading to accumulation of synovial fluid in the joint. Clinically, joint swelling is the predominant feature with associated pain and local tenderness.

Unlikely causes

Plantar fasciitis   The plantar fascia extends from the calcaneus (bone of the heel) to the middle phalanges of the toes. Patients will present with pain felt along the plantar surface of the foot and heel. Pain is insidious and progressively worsens. Runners are most prone to plantar fasciitis and may alter their running style to compensate for the pain.

Stress fractures of the elbow, knee and ankle   Clinical features will vary, depending on the cause and site of injury, but pain and marked tenderness should be present accompanied by swelling and some loss of function. Stress fractures are most commonly associated with the foot. Patients experience a dull ache along the affected metatarsal shaft, which changes to a sharp ache behind the metatarsal head.

189

Gout   Acute attacks of gout are exquisitely painful, with patients reporting that even bedclothes cannot be tolerated. Approximately 80% of cases affect the big toe. Gout is more prevalent in men, especially over the age of 50.

Repetitive strain injury   This condition, also called 'chronic upper limb pain syndrome', often results from prolonged periods of steady hand movement involving repeated grasping, turning and twisting. The predominant symptom is pain in all or one part of one or both arms. Usually, the person's job will involve repetitive tasks, such as keyboard operations.

Other causes of soft tissue injuries

Delayed onset muscle soreness This commonly follows unaccustomed strenuous activity, e.g. playing football for the first time in a long while or starting aerobic classes. Pain is felt in the muscles, which feel stiff and tight. Pain peaks within 72 hours. Patients should be encouraged to stretch properly before exercising to minimise the problem. No treatment is necessary.

Shin splint syndrome Recreational runners and people unaccustomed to regular running might experience pain along the front of the lower third of the tibia. Pressing gently on this area will cause considerable pain. It is caused by overstretching of the tibial muscle and is usually precipitated by running on hard surfaces. Pain is made worse by continued running or climbing stairs. Treatment involves running less frequently or for shorter distances and non-steroidal anti-inflammatory drug therapy for approximately 1 week.

Muscle strains Strains of the thigh muscles, either the quadriceps (front of the thigh) or hamstring (back of the thigh) are very common. Patients will not always be able to recall a specific event that has caused the strain. Pain and discomfort is worsened when the patient tries to use the muscle but daily activities can usually be performed.

190

TRIGGER POINTS indicative of referral: soft tissue injuries

- Acute injuries which show immediate swelling and severe pain.
- Children under 12 and elderly patients.
- Decreased range of motion in all direction involving the shoulder.
- Excessive range of movement in any joint (suggests major ligament disruption).
- Patients unable to bear any weight on an injured ankle/foot.
- Suspected fracture.
- Treatment failure.

Evidence of OTC medicine efficacy

Non-drug treatment plays a vital and major role in the treatment of soft tissue injuries. Standard advice follows the acronym RICE (Table 8.4).

Medication for soft tissue injuries is the same as for low back pain: systemic and topical analgesia.

Practical prescribing

Prescribing information relating to medication for soft tissue injuries is summarised in the appendix.

Table 8.4
Non-drug treatment of soft tissue injuries: RICE

Rest	● Allows immobilisation, enhancing healing and reducing blood flow
Ice	● Applied when the injury feels warm to the touch. Apply until the skin becomes numb and repeat at hourly intervals
Compression	● A crepe bandage provides a minimum level of compression. Avoid tubular stockings (e.g. Tubigrip) because they do not give adequate compression
Elevation	● Elevate the injury above the heart to help fluid drain away from the injury

Chapter 9

Paediatrics

Healthcare professionals are heavily dependent on getting details about the child's problem from the parents. Parents will know when their child is not well and asking about the child's general health will help to determine how poorly he or she actually is. As a general rule, any child that appears well can be managed by a nurse or pharmacist.

Head lice

Most children will experience head lice at some point. The lice can be transmitted only by prolonged head-to-head contact; fleeting contact will be insufficient for them to be transferred between heads.

Arriving at a differential diagnosis

Almost all parents will be seeking products to rid the child of head lice after self-diagnosis, or be concerned that their child has head lice because of a recent local outbreak at school. Occasionally, parents will also want to buy products to prevent their child contracting head lice. It is necessary to confirm the reasons for purchase and to eliminate dandruff or seborrhoeic dermatitis.

Clinical features of head lice

The presence of live lice is diagnostic. In addition, one-third of patients will experience scalp itching.

193

Conditions to eliminate

Unlikely causes

Dandruff Dandruff can cause irritation and itching of the scalp. The absence of live lice and the presence of skin flakes on the clothing should allow easy differentiation.

Seborrhoeic dermatitis Typically, seborrhoeic dermatitis will affect areas other than the scalp, most notably the face in adults and the napkin area in infants. In mild cases, if only the scalp is involved then the child might have persistent dandruff.

 TRIGGER POINTS indicative of referral: head lice

- Parents who find the cost of treatment prohibitive.

Evidence of OTC medicine efficacy

In the UK, OTC treatment primarily involves malathion, permethrin and phenothrin. Many trials have investigated the efficacy of insecticidal agents. An extensive review published by the Cochrane Library (Dodd, *Cochrane Review* 2000; issue 4) concluded that malathion and permethrin were effective, with high cure rates, but that insufficient evidence was available to demonstrate if one was more efficacious than the other. Unfortunately, these data were based on trials in which there was no prior exposure to the insecticides. It is well recognised that resistance to insecticides is seen in practice. To combat resistance, the current UK recommendation is based on a mosaic model, whereby the same product is used for a course of treatment (two applications 7 days apart). If this fails, another product from a different class should be tried.

Owing to the emerging problem of resistance, attention has focused on non-drug treatment options. The 'bug busting method' (wet combing) has received much attention. Current trial data clearly show bug busting to be less effective than insecticides (Roberts et al, *Lancet* 2000; 356: 540–544). Children are nearly three times as likely still to have head lice after bug busting than after using an insecticide, even in a geographical location known to have intermediate insecticidal resistance.

Practical prescribing

Prescribing information relating to head lice medication is summarised in the appendix.

HINTS AND TIPS

Who to treat?
No consensus opinion exists. In an ideal situation only patients with live lice should be treated. A more pragmatic approach is to treat all family members.

Application
Pay particular attention to the areas behind the ears and to the nape of the neck, as these areas are where lice are most often found.

Permethrin (Lyclear Creme Rinse)
One bottle is sufficient for shoulder-length hair of average thickness.

Phenothrin (Full Marks)
The lotion has to be left on 12 hours. For ease of use instruct parents to apply before bedtime and leave on overnight.

Lotion, liquid or shampoo?
- Shampoos do not work. The concentration of insecticide is too low to ensure eradication.
- Use liquid products for very young children and asthmatics.

Treatment failure
- Check for inappropriate usage and incorrect application before assuming that resistance is the cause.
- Patients should be told how best to check for infection. The easiest detection method is to comb damp or wet hair forward using a fine, metal-toothed comb (proprietary products are available and will remove even the smallest of newly hatched nymphs) over a pale or white piece of paper. If live lice are present then one or more will be visible on the paper.

Empty egg shells (nits)
- The presence of these does not constitute evidence of current infection. This is a common misconception held by the general public.
- Egg shells are not removed by using insecticides. Patients need to be reassured that the presence of egg shells does not mean treatment failure.

195

Threadworm (*Enterobius vermicularis*)

A social stigma surrounds the diagnosis of threadworm, with many patients believing that infection implies a lack of hygiene. This belief is unfounded as infection occurs in all social strata.

Arriving at a differential diagnosis

Threadworm should be one of the more simple conditions to diagnose. Patients generally present with very specific symptoms and very few other conditions need to be considered.

Probability	Cause
Most likely	Threadworm
Unlikely	Eczema/dermatitis
Very unlikely	Other worm infestations

Clinical features of threadworm

Night-time perianal itching is the classic presentation, and any child with these symptoms is almost certain to have threadworm. Itching can lead to sleep disturbances, resulting in irritability and tiredness the next day. Diagnosis can be confirmed by observing threadworm on the stool, although they are not always visible.

Conditions to eliminate

Unlikely causes

Eczema/dermatitis   No visible signs of infection or recent family history of threadworm could mean that the patient has dermatitis.

Very unlikely causes

Other worm infections   Roundworm and tapeworm infections are usually contracted when visiting poor or developing countries. A recent history of foreign travel can suggest these infections. Referral to the GP is needed.

> **!** TRIGGER POINTS indicative of referral: threadworm
>
> - Medication failure.
> - Secondary infection of perianal skin due to scratching.

Evidence of OTC medicine efficacy

Mebendazole and piperazine are available OTC. Mebendazole is certainly effective in roundworm infection but for other worm infections, including threadworm, the evidence is less clear with cure rates ranging from 60% to 82%.

Piperazine appears to be less effective than mebendazole. One comparison study found mebendazole to have a higher cure rate than piperazine (although the number of patients in the trial was low). The difference in cure rates might, in part, be due to their different mechanisms of action: mebendazole kills whereas piperazine paralyses threadworm. If paralysis wears off then the worm might be able to migrate back into the colon and thus treatment would fail.

Practical prescribing

Prescribing information relating to threadworm medication is summarised in the appendix.

HINTS AND TIPS

Who to treat?

- Treat all family members and not only the patient with symptoms, as it is likely that other family members will have been infected even though they do not show signs of infection.
- A repeated dose 14 days later is often recommended to ensure that worms maturing from ova at the time of the first dose are also eradicated.

Formulations

- Mebendazole (Ovex) can be chewed because it has been formulated to taste of orange.
- Piperazine elixir (Pripsen) is less convenient for patients because the manufacturers recommend that the dose is given for seven consecutive days.

Colic

There is no universally agreed definition of colic but the definition known as the 'rule of threes' is widely used. Thus, an infant could be considered to have colic if he or she cries for more than 3 hours a day for more than 3 days a week for more than 3 weeks. This definition does have its limitations, as few parents will wait 3 weeks to see if the infant meets the criteria. As a result, the third criterion is usually dropped in the clinical setting.

Arriving at a differential diagnosis

It is difficult to determine if a baby could be considered to have colic or is just crying excessively because the diagnosis of the condition depends on qualitative descriptions. Other conditions can cause prolonged crying and are listed below.

Probability	Cause
Most likely	Colic
Likely	Acute infection
Unlikely	Intolerance to cow's milk protein

Clinical features of colic

Besides obvious crying, the infant might show signs of abdominal pain, with a rigid abdomen, the legs drawn up towards the chest and the fists clenched. Pain might be mild, causing the child to be restless, or severe, resulting in rhythmical screaming attacks. These tend to last a few minutes at a time, alternating with equally long quiet periods in which the child almost goes to sleep.

Conditions to eliminate

Likely causes

Acute infection   Colic and acute infections of the ear or urinary tract can present with almost identical symptoms. However, it is unusual for children with an acute infection

198

to have a previous history of excessive crying and they should also show signs of systemic infection, such as fever.

Unlikely causes

Intolerance to cow's milk protein   Colicky pain in infants is sometimes due to intolerance to cow's milk protein. This is far less common than generally believed but should be considered if the infant is not putting on weight as expected.

 TRIGGER POINTS indicative of referral: colic

- Infants that are failing to put on weight.
- Medication failure.
- Overanxious parents.

Evidence of OTC medicine efficacy

Dimethicone (simethicone) is reported to have antifoaming properties, reducing surface tension and allowing easier elimination of gas from the gut by passing flatus or belching. It is widely used yet no evidence of its efficacy exists. It might be a useful placebo for anxious and often tired and irritable parents who want to give their baby some form of medication.

Practical prescribing

Prescribing information relating to colic medication is summarised in the appendix.

HINTS AND TIPS

- Review feeding technique (for bottle-fed babies): before recommending a product it is worth checking feeding technique. Underfeeding a baby can result in excessive sucking, which results in air being swallowed leading to colic-like symptoms. Additionally, the teat size of the bottle should be checked. If correct, when the bottle is turned upside down the milk should drop slowly from the bottle.

Atopic dermatitis

Atopic dermatitis is an allergic skin condition that mainly affects infants and young children, with the majority of patients growing out of the condition by their early teens. Approximately 60% of children will develop atopic dermatitis within the first year and there appears to be a genetic link.

Arriving at a differential diagnosis

The most likely cause of itchy skin in children under 2 years old seen in primary care is atopic dermatitis, especially if there is a family or personal history of atopy. Practitioners should therefore direct questions to confirm this diagnosis as other causes of skin rashes affect this age group and are listed below.

Probability	Cause
Most likely	Atopic dermatitis
Likely	Seborrhoeic dermatitis, contact dermatitis
Unlikely	Psoriasis

Clinical features of atopic dermatitis

A typical presentation is an irritable, scratching child with dermatitis of varying severity. The child might have had the symptoms for some time and the parent has often already tried some form of cream to help control the itch and rash (Fig. 9.1).

Table 9.1 lists some of the questions that should be asked to aid diagnosis.

Conditions to eliminate

Likely causes

Seborrhoeic dermatitis Seborrhoeic dermatitis typically occurs in the first 6 months. It usually affects the scalp (where large yellow scales and crusts often appear), face and napkin area. Itching is generally not present. The condition usually resolves and spontaneously seldom recurs.

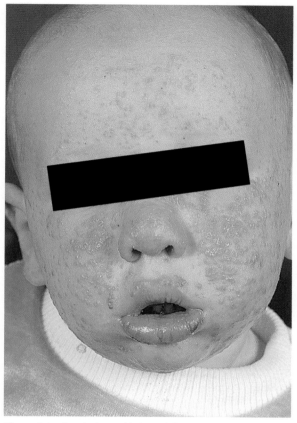

Figure 9.1 Atopic dermatitis in an infant. Reproduced from *Dermatology: An Illustrated Colour Text* by D Gawkrodger, 2002, Mosby, with permission.

Contact dermatitis Lesions will itch and appear red or brown. Itching is a prominent feature and often causes the patient to scratch, resulting in broken and weeping skin. The longer the condition persists, the more likely that dryness and scaling of the skin is seen. The rash might have an identifiable cause, e.g. reaction to sensitising agents in soap or perfumes.

Table 9.1
Specific questions to ask the patient: atopic dermatitis

Question	Relevance
Is itching present?	● Intense itching suggests atopic dermatitis ● Rashes that do not itch suggest psoriasis and seborrhoeic dermatitis
Distribution of rash	● An affected nappy area suggests seborrhoeic dermatitis ● A clear nappy area suggests atopic dermatitis ● In babies, cheeks, wrists and hand involvement suggests atopic dermatitis ● In toddlers and older children, behind the knee, in front or at the bend of the elbow and ankles suggests atopic dermatitis
Family history of atopy	● If a parent has eczema, hay fever or asthma then atopic dermatitis is likely

Unlikely causes

Psoriasis   Psoriasis in older children often affects similar parts of the body as atopic dermatitis and can therefore be confused. However, the rash in psoriasis tends to be raised, with well-defined boundaries and a silvery-white scaly appearance; itch, if present, is mild.

TRIGGER POINTS indicative of referral: atopic dermatitis

● Children with widespread or severe dermatitis.
● Medication failure.
● Presence of secondary infection (weeping and crusting lesions).

HINTS AND TIPS

● Baths: patients should be told to have lukewarm, not hot, baths because hot water can aggravate the problem. In addition, a bath additive should be used (e.g. Balneum, Oilatum, Emulsiderm) to help hydration of the skin.

Evidence of OTC medicine efficacy

OTC management for atopic dermatitis consists of avoiding potential irritants, managing dry skin and controlling itching. OTC topical steroids are licensed only for children > 10 years, which limits their usefulness. Management does not appear to be based on evidence but on clinical experience and common sense.

Avoiding irritants

The use of highly perfumed soaps and detergents should be discouraged and soap substitutes should be used (e.g. Alpha Keri, Neutrogena).

Emollients

None of the published literature appears to have addressed whether one emollient is superior to another. Patients might have to try several emollients before finding one that is most effective for their skin.

Antihistamines

There appear to be no clinical trial data on the use of sedative antihistamines for reducing pruritus in atopic dermatitis, but they are often prescribed to children to prevent scratching at night.

Practical prescribing

Prescribing information relating to medication for atopic dermatitis is summarised in the appendix.

203

Fever

Normal oral temperature is 37°C (98.6°F), plus or minus 1°C. Above these limits the person is said to have a fever. Fever is a common symptom of many conditions and is therefore extremely common.

Arriving at a differential diagnosis

The most likely cause of fever seen in primary care will be viral infection. Practitioners should therefore direct questions to confirm this diagnosis as other causes of fever are seen in primary care and listed below.

Probability	Cause
Most likely	Upper respiratory tract infection (mainly viral)
Likely	Urinary tract infection
Unlikely	Medicine-induced fever
Very unlikely	Meningitis, glandular fever, sixth disease

Clinical features of fever

Children with fever will generally be irritable and off their food and will seek more parental attention than usual. In many cases, the parent will not actually have measured the temperature and will have diagnosed fever based on subjective perception. Depending on the cause of fever, the child might exhibit other symptoms such as cold, cough, sore throat and earache, for example if fever is caused by an upper respiratory tract infection. Table 9.2 lists some of the questions that should be asked to aid diagnosis.

Conditions to eliminate

Likely causes

Urinary tract infection   Children under 2 years of age with a urinary tract infection will present with fever and very few other diagnostic symptoms. Diarrhoea, irritability and loss of appetite can occur but are also present with other infections. Children older than 2 years, especially girls, may show cystitis-like symptoms.

Table 9.2
Specific questions to ask the patient: fever

Question	Relevance
How poorly is the child?	● The parent will know how poorly the child is relative to normal behaviour. This can be more important than the height of the fever, e.g. a child can have a high temperature but be relatively normal whereas a child with a mild temperature might be quite poorly
Associated symptoms	● Cough, cold and sore throat suggest upper respiratory tract infection ● Fatigue and lymph node enlargement in teenagers suggest glandular fever ● Fever alone suggests a urinary tract infection

Unlikely causes

Medicine-induced fever A number of medicines can elevate body temperature and should be considered if no other cause can be determined. Penicillins, cephalosporins, macrolides, tricyclic antidepressants, anticonvulsants and anti-inflammatory medicines have all been associated with increasing temperature.

Very unlikely causes

Glandular fever This is most commonly seen in patients aged 15–24, is rare in children under 5 and is less frequent in those aged 5–14. Symptoms are vague but characterised by low fever (< 38.5°C), fatigue, headache, sore throat and swollen and tender lymph glands. The symptoms tend to be mild but can linger for many months.

Meningitis Signs and symptoms are non-specific in the early stages of the disease and include fever, nausea, vomiting, headache and irritability. Symptoms can develop quickly and be unpredictable, especially in infants and young children. Fever, lethargy, vomiting and irritability are common in children aged between 3 months and 2 years, and severe headache, stiff neck and photophobia are more common in older children and adults. In the later stages of the disease a petechial or purpuric non-blanching rash characteristically develops in meningococcal infection.

Roseola infantum (sixth disease) Roseola infantum is most prevalent in children under 1 year of age. Onset is with a sudden high fever (40°C) that usually subsides by the third or fourth day once the rash, which blanches when pressed, appears on the trunk and limbs. The condition is self-limiting and referral is not usually necessary.

> **❗ TRIGGER POINTS indicative of referral: fever**
>
> - Any feverish child under 3 months old.
> - Fever accompanied with no other symptoms.
> - If the patient has suffered any febrile convulsion.
> - Purpuric rash.
> - Stiff neck.

Evidence of OTC medicine efficacy

Paracetamol and ibuprofen have proven efficacy as antipyretics and both can be used to reduce temperature. However, there is a lack of evidence to show that combinations of both, or alternating paracetamol and ibuprofen, are better than using a single agent.

Practical prescribing

Prescribing information relating to medication for fever is summarised in the appendix.

HINTS AND TIPS

Taking a temperature
- If using a mercury thermometer, shake the thermometer before use.
- When taking an oral temperature the thermometer should be placed under the tongue for 2–3 minutes. Before the temperature is taken it is important to wait at least 10 minutes after eating anything hot or cold.

Drinking fluids
Children should be encouraged to drink additional fluid to prevent dehydration, as a fever will make them sweat more than usual.

Chapter 10

Specific product requests

Many patients will directly ask for advice on named medicines, or will want to purchase them. This chapter deals with those situations in which patients ask for a particular product but require some level of assessment by a healthcare professional before the request can be complied with.

Motion sickness

Motion sickness can affect any individual in any form of moving vehicle and is characterised by nausea, pallor and occasionally vomiting. Children between 2 and 12 years are most commonly affected, although certain occupations, e.g. naval crew and pilots, also show a higher prevalence rate than the normal population. It is widely believed that motion sickness results from the brain's inability to process conflicting information received from sensory nerve terminals concerning movement and position, the eyes and the vestibular system of the ear.

Evidence of OTC medicine efficacy

First-generation antihistamines (cyclizine, cinnarizine, meclozine and promethazine) and the anticholinergic hyoscine are routinely recommended to prevent motion sickness. All have shown various degrees of effectiveness, with hyoscine consistently proving the most effective. On this basis hyoscine-containing products should be used first line.

Non-pharmacological approaches to the prevention of motion sickness using acupressure are also available OTC. Bruce et al (*Aviation Space and Environmental Medicine* 1990; 61: 361–365) investigated the use of Sea Band acupressure bands compared with hyoscine and placebo. Eighteen healthy volunteers were subjected to simulated conditions to induce motion sickness. The findings showed that, whereas hyoscine exerted a preventative effect, Sea Bands were no more effective than placebo. Further trials have confirmed these findings, although a small trial by Stern et al (*Alternative Therapy and Health Medicine* 1992; 7: 91–4) reported positive findings. Further trials are needed because acupressure has shown positive effects for nausea and vomiting associated with pregnancy.

Practical prescribing

Proscribing information relating to medication for motion sickness is summarised in the appendix.

Dosing for each medicine is shown in Table 10.1, and further prescribing information relating to medication for motion sickness is summarised in the appendix.

HINTS AND TIPS

Product selection should be based on matching up the length of the journey with the duration of action of each medicine:

- journeys of up to 4 hours: recommend hyoscine
- journeys 4–8 hours long: recommend cinnarizine
- journeys over 8 hours: recommend promethazine and meclozine.

Dry mouth problems
Many people will complain of a dry mouth with travel sickness medicines. This is easily overcome by telling the patient to suck a sweet.

Emergency hormonal contraception (EHC)

In January 2001, emergency hormonal contraception became available to the public without a prescription through community pharmacies, either as a direct purchase or through a patient group direction. The product contains two levonorgestrel 0.75-mg tablets and is marketed under the name of Levonelle. The exact mechanism of action for levonorgestrel is not clear but it is thought to work mainly by preventing ovulation and fertilisation by causing endometrial changes that discourage egg implantation.

Table 10.1
Prescribing information for medication for motion sickness

Medicine	Dosage	Notes
Cyclizine (Valoid)	> 6 years: half a tablet three times a day > 12 years: one tablet three times a day	Subject to abuse and rarely stocked/ given out by pharmacies
Cinnarizine (Stugeron)	5–12 years: one tablet, repeat every 8 hours if needed > 12 years: two tablets, repeat every 8 hours if needed	Take 2 hours before travelling
Meclozine (Sea-Legs)	2–6 years: half a tablet 6–12 years: one tablet > 12 years: two tablets	Take 1 hour before travelling
Promethazine (Avomine)	5–10 years: half a tablet > 10 years: one tablet	Take 2 hours before travelling
Hyoscine (Joy-Rides)	3–4 years: half a tablet (max. one in 24 hours) 4–7 years: one tablet (max. two in 24 hours) 7–12 years: 1–2 tablets	Take 20–30 minutes before travelling
Junior Kwells	4–10 years: half to one tablet	
Kwells	10–12 years: half to one tablet Adults: one tablet	

Evidence of OTC medicine efficacy

The exact effectiveness of Levonelle is hard to establish, as many people who have been treated with emergency contraception would not have become pregnant even without treatment. However, when Levonelle was compared against the Yuzpe regimen (Schering PC4), the progestogen-only regimen was found to prevent 86% of expected pregnancies when treatment was initiated within 72 hours, compared with 57% with PC4. Levonorgestrel is more effective the earlier it is taken after unprotected sex:

- 95% of pregnancies are prevented if taken within 24 hours
- 85% of pregnancies are prevented if taken between 24 and 48 hours
- 58% of pregnancies are prevented if taken between 48 and 72 hours.

Practical prescribing and product selection

Assessing patient suitability

Prior to any sale/supply of Levonelle, an assessment has to be made on the likelihood that the patient is pregnant. Ask:

1. Has the patient had unprotected sex, contraceptive failure or missed taking contraceptive pills in the last 24 hours? Emergency hormonal contraception can be given only to patients who present within 72 hours. If more than 72 hours but less than 120 hours (5 days) has elapsed, the patient can have an intrauterine device fitted.
2. Is the patient already pregnant? Details about the patient's last period should be sought. Is the period late? If so, how many days late? Was the nature of the period different or unusual. If pregnancy is suspected, a pregnancy test could be offered.
3. What method of contraception is normally used? Patients who take combined oral contraceptives might not need emergency hormonal contraception, depending on when in the cycle the pill was forgotten. The Royal College of Obstetricians and Gynaecologists' guidelines on missed pills is:
   - If two or more pills are missed from the first seven pills in a packet or four or more pills are missed mid-packet then emergency hormonal contraception should be given.
   - If two or more pills are missed from the last seven pills in a packet, emergency hormonal contraception is not needed providing the pill-free break is omitted.
   - If the patient uses a progestogen-only form of contraception then emergency hormonal contraception should always be given if the tablet is taken more than 3 hours late.

HINTS AND TIPS

- Who is eligible? Only patients over the age of 16 can be sold Levonelle, although family planning services, GPs and pharmacists acting under a patient group direction can supply emergency hormonal contraception to patients under 16. Patient group directions for Levonelle can be accessed online at www.druginfozone.nhs.uk/pgd/DisplayProtocolsInDrugName.asp?ID=296

- Do you have to supply emergency hormonal contraception? The supply of emergency hormonal contraception is at the discretion of each practitioner and some, for religious beliefs, might choose not to supply emergency hormonal contraception. However, the patient must be advised on other local sources of supply so that she can access the service.

- Taking EHC may affect the timing of the next period; it might be earlier or later than usual.

- If the period is different from normal or >5 days late then a pregnancy test could be offered.

- About one in five patients experiences nausea but only 1 in 20 goes on to vomit. If the patient vomits within 3 hours of the dose she should be advised to obtain a further supply of EHC.

- A number of medicines interfere with Levonelle absorption (appendix), reducing its effectiveness. Such cases are best referred to the GP. Doubling the dose of Levonelle is commonly practised (though not licensed).

Prescribing information relating to Levonelle is summarised in the appendix.

Nicotine replacement therapy (NRT)

Smoking represents the single greatest cause of preventable illness and premature death worldwide. According to UK government figures for 2002, 26% of the adult population smoke. Smoking is responsible for or contributes to a myriad of conditions, including lung cancer, ischaemic heart disease and chronic obstructive pulmonary disease. Three compounds in cigarettes are of real clinical importance: (i) tar-based products, which have carcinogenic properties; (ii) carbon monoxide, which reduces the oxygen-carrying capacity of the red blood cells; and (iii) nicotine, which produces dependence.

Evidence of OTC medicine efficacy

Nicotine replacement therapy has established itself as an effective treatment option. Numerous well-designed clinical trials have shown that nicotine replacement therapy doubles the success rate of those attempting to stop smoking compared with placebo. There are a number of drug delivery systems, all of which have been shown to be more effective than placebo. Comparative trials between delivery systems appear not to have been conducted so is not possible to say if one delivery system is better than another. Patient preference will be the determining factor in which system is chosen.

Practical prescribing

In 1998, evidence-based smoking cessation guidelines were produced by the Health Education Authority and published in the journal *Thorax*. These guidelines recommended the use of nicotine replacement therapy and advocated that health-care professionals must give smokers accurate information on nicotine replacement therapy products.

Prior to instigation of any treatment it is important that the patient does want to stop smoking. Work has shown that motivation is a major determinant for successful smoking cessation and interventions based on the transtheoretical model of change have proved effective (Fig. 10.1). This model identifies six stages, progress through which is cyclical and patients need varying types of support and advice at each stage.

Most patients who ask directly for nicotine replacement therapy will be at the preparation stage of the model and ready to enter the action stage. However, a small number of patients might well be buying nicotine replacement therapy to please others and are actually in the precontemplation stage and do not want to stop smoking.

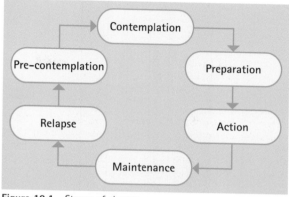

Figure 10.1 Stages of change.

Suitability of nicotine replacement therapy preparations

All patients, providing they are over 18 years old, can use nicotine replacement therapy, except if they are pregnant or are breastfeeding. Nicotine replacement therapy is not contraindicated in patients with pre-existing heart disease, and research has shown that nicotine replacement therapy can be safely given in this patient group, although product licences for OTC products state that they should not be given. In practice, it would not seem unreasonable to allow these patients to use nicotine replacement therapy, although it might be prudent to speak first with the patient's GP. Side-effects with nicotine replacement therapy are rare and are normally limited to either gastrointestinal problems associated with accidental ingestion of nicotine when chewing gum or local skin irritation and vivid dreams associated with patches. Headache, nausea and diarrhoea have also been reported. Nicotine replacement therapy also appears not to have any significant interactions with other medicines.

Nicotine replacement therapy is formulated as gum, lozenges, patches, nasal spray, inhalator and sublingual tablets. Table 10.2 lists the delivery routes for each of the branded products available OTC.

215

Table 10.2
Delivery routes for the branded nicotine replacement therapy products available OTC

Name	Gum	Lozenge	Patch	Spray	Inhalator	Microtab
Nicorette	✓		✓	✓	✓	✓
Nicotinell	✓	✓	✓			
NiQuitin CQ	✓	✓	✓			

Nicotine gum

Nicotine gum is flavoured (citrus, mint or fruit) because unflavoured gum can leave a bitter taste. Nicotine gum should be chewed slowly until the taste becomes strong; it should then be rested between the cheek and gum until the taste fades, when it can then be re-chewed. Each piece of nicotine gum lasts approximately 30 minutes.

It should take approximately 3 months to break the habit of smoking, after which the nicotine gum should be gradually used less often. When daily use is one or two pieces of gum the patient should be told to stop using it.

Nicotine patches

Patches deliver a constant level of nicotine over a 16- or 24-hour period. Nicotinell and Niquitin CQ patches are worn continuously and changed every 24 hours and are suitable for those smokers who need a cigarette as soon as they wake up. Vivid dreams have been reported as a side-effect in approximately 5% of users and may be due to the circulating nicotine levels.

Patches should be to non-hairy skin on the trunk or upper arm, but the same area should be avoided on consecutive days as local skin reactions are reported in around 30% of patients.

Nicotine lozenges

The patient should be instructed to suck one lozenge every 1–2 hours when they have the urge to smoke. The usual dosage is 8–12 lozenges per day. Lozenges are used in a similar way to the gum:

1. Suck until the taste becomes strong.
2. The lozenge should then be lodged between the gum and cheek.
3. When the taste fades, begin to suck the lozenge again.
4. Each lozenge lasts approximately 30 minutes.

Nicotine inhalation cartridge

The inhaler is of particular benefit to those smokers who still feel they need to continue the hand-to-mouth movement. Each cartridge is inserted into the inhaler and air is drawn into the mouth through the mouthpiece. Deep

---

HINTS AND TIPS

16- or 24-hour patches?
- A 16-hour patch will be suitable for most patients. However, if a patient requires a cigarette within the first 20–30 minutes after waking then a 24-hour patch should be given.
- If sleep disturbances are experienced with the 24-hour patches patients can switch to a 16-hour patch or, alternatively, remove the 24-hour patch when they go to bed.

---

drawing or short sucking can be used as required by the individual. Each cartridge lasts about 20 minutes.

Microtabs

Microtabs are delivered sublingually and patients should be instructed to place the tablet under the tongue. Patients who smoke fewer than 20 cigarettes a day can increase the dosage to that recommended for smokers who smoke more than 20 cigarettes a day if the one tablet per hour regimen fails or if the nicotine withdrawal symptoms remain so strong they believe they will relapse. Most patients need between 8 and 24 tablets a day, although the maximum is 40 tablets in 24 hours.

Spray

A further delivery route is intranasally. It is important to instruct the patient on its correct use:

1. Remove the protective cap.
2. Prime the device if using the spray for the first time or if you have not used the spray for 2–3 days. This is done by pressing the bottle several times until a fine spray appears.
3. Insert the spray tip into one nostril, pointing the top towards the back of the nose.
4. Press firmly and quickly.
5. Repeat in to the other nostril.
6. Replace cap.

Table 10.3 summarises the prescribing data for all products.

Table 10.3
Nicotine replacement therapy prescribing data

Medicine	Dosage
Nicorette Gum	• 20 cigarettes: one piece (4 mg) of gum chewed when urge to smoke; max. 15 in 24 hours • < 20 cigarettes: one piece (2 mg) of gum chewed when urge to smoke; max. 15 in 24 hours
Nicotinell Gum	• 20 cigarettes: one piece (4 mg) of gum chewed when urge to smoke; max. 25 in 24 hours • < 20 cigarettes: one piece (2 mg) of gum chewed when urge to smoke; max. 25 in 24 hours
NiQuitin CQ Gum	• Urge to smoke first cigarette within 30 minutes of getting up: one piece (4 mg) of gum chewed when urge to smoke; max. 15 in 24 hours
Nicorette Patches	• > 20 cigarettes: 15 mg for 8 weeks; 10 mg for 2 weeks; 5 mg for 2 weeks
Nicotinell Patches	• 20 cigarettes: TTS 30 (21 mg) for 3–4 weeks; TTS 20 (14 mg) for 3–4 weeks; TTS 10 (7 mg) for 3–4 weeks • < 20 cigarettes: TTS 20 (14 mg) for 3–4 weeks; TTS 10 (7 mg) for 3–4 weeks
NiQuitin CQ	• 10 cigarettes: 21 mg for 6 weeks; 14 mg for 2 weeks; 7 mg × for 2 weeks • < 10 cigarettes: 14 mg for 6 weeks; 7 mg for 2 weeks
Nicotinell Lozenge	• 30 cigarettes: one (4-mg) lozenge every 1–2 hours; max. 15 in 24 hours • < 30 cigarettes: one (2-mg) lozenge every 1–2 hours; max. 30 in 24 hours • Manufacturer's recommended dose is tailored to individual patient response

219

table continues

Table 10.3 continued

Medicine	Dosage
NiQuitin CQ Lozenge	• Urge to smoke first cigarette within 30 minutes of getting up: use 4-mg lozenge; all other patients use 2-mg lozenges • One lozenge every 1–2 hours for 6 weeks • One lozenge every 2–4 hours for 3 weeks • One lozenge every 4–8 hours for 3 weeks • One lozenge once or twice daily for 12 weeks
Nicorette inhalator	• Manufacturer does not make a distinction between the number of cigarettes smoked and the dosing: • 6–12 cartridges for 8 weeks • 3–6 cartridges for 2 weeks • Reduce to zero for 2 weeks
Nicorette Microtabs	• >20 cigarettes: two tablets (4 mg) every hour for 12 weeks • < 20 cigarettes: one tablet (2 mg) every hour for 12 weeks
Nicorette Spray	• Manufacturer does not make a distinction between the number of cigarettes smoked and the dosing: one spray into each nostril up to twice per hour for 8 weeks; max 64 sprays in 24 hours. Over the next 2 weeks reduce dose by half and the last 2 weeks reduce to zero

Malaria prophylaxis

Background

Malaria is a parasitic disease spread by the female *Anopheles* mosquito. Four species of protozoon produce malaria in humans: *Plasmodium vivax*, *P. ovale*, *P. malariae* and *P.*

falciparum. Malaria is a leading cause of death in areas of the world where the infection is endemic, with an estimated 300 million cases each year resulting in over 1 million deaths. However, malaria is not only confined to endemic malarial areas and the number of cases reported in Western countries is on the increase. The risk of contracting malaria varies greatly and depends on the area visited, the time of year and altitude. In general, risk tends to increase in more remote areas compared with urban/tourist areas, after rainy or monsoon seasons and at low altitude.

P. falciparum is the most virulent form of malaria and is responsible for the majority of deaths associated with malaria infection.

Clinically the patient suffers from chills, nausea, vomiting and headache. This is followed by fever, which concludes with sweating. This cycle repeats every 2–3 days.

Evidence of OTC medicine efficacy

Antimalarial medication should be taken in all areas where the threat of malaria exists. Chloroquine and proguanil are available OTC and have proven efficacy.

Unfortunately, widespread resistance to these two medicines now limits their usefulness. Always check current guidance for the destination the client is travelling to or through. In most instances, *MIMS* would be a first-line reference source as guidance is updated monthly (unlike the *BNF*, which is produced every 6 months).

Practical prescribing

Chloroquine (e.g. Avloclor, Nivaquine)

Chloroquine can be given alone or in combination with proguanil and is restricted to areas in which the risk of chloroquine-resistant falciparum malaria is still low, such as the Indian subcontinent. Adults and children over 13 should take 300 mg of chloroquine base each week, which is equivalent to two tablets, e.g. Avloclor contains chloroquine phosphate 250 mg, which is equivalent to 155 mg of chloroquine base per tablet; Nivaquine contains chloroquine sulphate 200 mg, which is equivalent to 150 mg of chloroquine base.

A syrup formulation of Nivaquine is available (50 mg of base/5 mL) and should be recommended to children because

HINTS AND TIPS

Avoid being bitten by:

- using an insecticide, particularly one containing diethyl toluamide (DEET)
- wearing long-sleeved shirts and trousers, especially at dawn and dusk.
- checking hotel windows to make sure they have adequate screening
- sleeping under a mosquito net
- keeping doors and windows closed during the evening and night
- using mosquito coils or plug-in dispensers.

Antimalarials need to be taken before (at least 1 week), during and after (4 weeks) visiting a malaria endemic region. Taking the medication prior to departure allows patients to know if they are going to experience side-effects and, if they do, have time to obtain a different antimalarial. It also helps to establish a medicine-taking routine, which might help with compliance. Continuing medication for 4 weeks after leaving the region ensures that any possible infection that could have been contracted on the final days of the stay does not develop into malaria.

Application of DEET
- The concentration of DEET in commercial products varies widely. Products with concentrations in excess of 50% can cause skin irritation and occasionally skin blistering. It is advisable that these are patch-tested first before widespread application.
- DEET should be reapplied every 3–4 hours to ensure adequate protection.
- DEET can damage certain plastics, e.g. sunglasses. It is important to emphasise that clients wash their hands after applying DEET.

Illness on return from malarial region
- Patients should be told to report flu-like symptoms to their GP for 3 months after returning from holiday.

222

an accurate dose can be given according to their weight. Patients with psoriasis might notice a worsening of their condition.

Proguanil (Paludrine)

Proguanil is always used in combination with chloroquine. A problem with dosing regimens involving proguanil is that it has to be taken daily in addition to weekly taking of chloroquine.

Prescribing information relating to antimalarials is summarised in the appendix.

Sunburn

Rays from the ultraviolet (UV) region of the light spectrum are responsible for suntan and sunburn; UVA is responsible for causing skin tanning and UVB for sunburn. The body's response to the effects of UVA and UVB light is protective. Melanin production increases, causing a darkening of the skin, the all-important suntan. Unfortunately, melanin synthesis is slow and skin damage might well have already occurred (sunburn). The consequences of skin damage can lead to carcinoma and the incidence of sun-related cancers is on the increase, especially in white-skinned people living in equatorial regions.

Evidence of OTC medicine efficacy

Very few medicines offer a specific treatment for sunburn; prevention is truly better than cure. Sunscreens filter UVA and UVB, preventing burning and premature ageing of skin. The sun protection factor (SPF) gives a rough estimate of the efficiency of the product to block UVB. For example, if a person normally shows signs of burning in 30 minutes without protection, a product with an SPF of 6 would extend the period of time by six times, so that burning would begin at 3 hours.

Practical prescribing and product selection

Current recommendations advocate that all white-skinned people should use a sunscreen with an SPF of 15. This level of protection is effectively a sun block because it absorbs more than 90% of UV radiation and, provided it is applied in sufficient quantity and regularly (every 2–3 hours), then higher SPF sunscreens are not needed. Chemical and physical sunscreens are available, although chemical sunscreens are often preferred as they are cosmetically more acceptable as they rub in to the skin compared to physical sunscreens, which provide an opaque barrier to UV light.

HINTS AND TIPS

How to avoid sunburn
- Sunburn can occur on cloudy days because UV light is not effectively filtered by cloud cover. Patients should therefore still apply sunscreen.
- Try to be indoors during the hottest part of the day (between 10.00 a.m. and 2.00 p.m.).
- Wear a hat with a brim and long-sleeved shirts and trousers during the hottest part of the day.

Water-resistant sunscreens
- These are not truly water resistant. It would be prudent to reapply sunscreens after swimming.

Eye protection
- Wear wrap-around sunglasses: prolonged (over years) sun exposure can lead contribute to age-related macular degeneration.

Medicine-induced photosensitivity
- Piroxicam, tetracyclines, chlorpromazine, phenothiazines and amiodarone can cause pruritus and skin rash when the skin is exposed to natural sunlight.

Practical prescribing: summary of medicines

Condition	Treatment	Dosing	Likely side-effects	Significant interactions	Care needed
Acne vulgaris	First line	Benzoyl peroxide	> 12 years: apply twice daily	Skin irritation, burning or peeling	--------None--------
Atopic dermatitis	First line	Emollients	Birth onwards: apply prn	None, although some products contain sensitising excipients (see *BNF* section 13.1.3)	--------None--------
	Second line	Antihistamines, e.g. chlorphenamine (Piriton) syrup	1-2 years: 1 mg (2.5 mL) bd 2-6 years: 1 mg (2.5 mL) tds/qds 6-12 years: 2 mg (5 mL) tds/qds Note: A number of alternative antihistamines could be tried, e.g. azatadine (Optimine), brompheniramine (Dimotane), clemastine (Tavegil), cyproheptadine (Periactin), promethazine (Phenergan)	Sedation, dry mouth	Increased sedation with opioid analgesics, hypnotics and antidepressants, although it is unlikely that children will be taking such medicines	None

table continues

Appendix continued

Condition	Treatment	Dosing	Likely side-effects	Significant interactions	Care needed
Back pain	First line: systemic	Ibuprofen Systemic: > 12 years: 200–400 mg tds	Gastrointestinal effects, e.g. nausea and diarrhoea Topical formulations can cause skin rash	Lithium, anticoagualants, methotrexate	Avoid in pregnancy and breast feeding, and in patients with moderate/severe renal impairment and with a history of peptic ulcer Care in asthmatics and in mild renal impairment: use lowest effective dose
	Second line: systemic	Paracetamol > 12 years: 500–1000 mg qds prn	----------------None----------------		Avoid large doses in liver disease, e.g. alcoholics

	First line: topical (if systemic not applicable)	NSAIDs (e.g. ibuprofen, piroxicam, diclofenac ketoprofen, felbinac)	> 12 years: apply three or four times a day	--------None--------
	Second line: topical	Rubefacients	> 5/6 years: prn up to four times a day	Local irritation	--------None--------
Blepharitis	First line	Maintain lid hygiene	Apply mild (baby shampoo) with a cotton bud	--------Not applicable--------
	Second line	Warm compress	Apply for 10–20 minutes twice a day	--------Not applicable--------
Cold sores	First line	Aciclovir (e.g. Soothelip, Virasorb, Zovirax)	> 12 years: apply five times a day	Stinging	Avoid in immunocom- promised patients
	Second line	Products containing anaesthetics (e.g. lidocaine as Lypsyl cold sore gel)	> 12 years: apply three or four times a day	Stinging	None (although manufacturers advise caution in pregnancy)

table continues

227

Appendix continued

Condition	Treatment		Dosing	Likely side-effects	Significant interactions	Care needed
	Second line	Products containing analgesics (e.g Bonjela)	No lower age limit: apply every 3 hours		----None----	
Colic	First line	Dimethicone (e.g. Infacol, Dentinox)	Birth upwards: 20–40 mg after each feed. Note: Proprietary products vary in their mg/mL strength and therefore volume given to child will vary		----None----	
Conjunctivitis – allergic	First line	Allergen avoidance		----Not applicable----		
	First line medication	Levocabastine	> 12 years: one drop bd into both eyes	Local irritation, blurred vision	----None----	
	Second line medication	Sodium cromoglicate	No lower age limit: one or two drops qds into both eyes	Local irritation, blurred vision	----None----	
Conjunctivitis – bacterial	First line	Propamidine	No lower age limit: one or two drops qds. Apply od/bd for ointment	Blurred vision	----None----	

228

Constipation	First line	Increase fibre	------------------------Not applicable------------------------		
	Second line (any laxative)	Bulk-forming (e.g. Fybogel)	6–12 years: 2.5–5 mL bd > 12 years: one sachet bd Note: Other bulk-forming laxatives are available, e.g. methylcellulose (Celevac), sterculia (Normacol)	Flatulence and abdominal pain	None	Avoid in patients with faecal impaction and ensure all patients maintain adequate fluid intake
	Second line	Stimulant (e.g. senna)	6–12 years: 7.5–15 mg (5–10 mL) od > 12 years: 15–30 mg (2–4 tablets) od Note: Other stimulant laxatives are available, e.g. glycerol, bisacodyl (Dulcolax), sodium picosulphate (Laxoberal)	Abdominal pain	------------------None------------------	
	Second line	Osmotic (e.g. lactulose)	< 1 year: 2.5 mL bd 1–5 years: 5 mL bd 5–10 years: 10 mL bd > 10 years: 15 mL bd	Flatulence, abdominal pain and colic	------------------None------------------	

table continues

Appendix continued

Condition	Treatment	Dosing	Likely side-effects	Significant interactions	Care needed
	Second line	Stool softener (e.g. docusate)	Note: other osmotic laxatives are available, e.g. lactitol, magnesium hydroxide	None reported	--------None--------
			6 months–2 years: 12.5 mg (5 mL paed. sol.) tds		
			2–12 years: 12.5–25 mg (5–10 mL) tds		
			Adults: up to 500 mg in divided doses		
Corns and calluses	First line	Relieve pressure	--------Not applicable--------		
	Second line	Salicylic acid	> 6 years: apply od	Local skin irritation	None	Avoid in diabetics
			Note: Corns/calluses rare in children			
Common cold	First line	Decongestants (e.g. pseudoephedrine)	> 1 year: 11.25 mg qds*	Insomnia most likely	Avoid with monoamine oxidase inhibitors, moclobemide, beta-blockers	Avoid in first trimester of pregnancy and severe renal impairment
			6–12 years: 30 mg (half a tablet) qds	Might cause tachycardia		
			> 12 years: 60 mg (one tablet) qds			

*relates to Tixycolds syrup

		Dose	Side effects	Interactions	Cautions
Second line	Chlorphenamine (e.g. Piriton)	1–2 years: 1 mg (2.5 mL) bd 2–6 years: 1 mg (2.5 mL) tds/qds 6–12 years: 2 mg (5 mL) tds/qds	Sedation, dry mouth, constipation	sibutramine and tricyclic antidepressants Increased sedation with opioid analgesics, anxiolytics, hypnotics and antidepressants	Caution in patients with glaucoma and prostate enlargement Appears safe in pregnancy but some manufacturers advise avoidance
Cough – productive First line	Increase fluid intake	----------Not applicable----------		----------None----------	
Second line	Guaifenesin	1–6 years: 50 mg qds 6–12 years: 100 mg qds > 12 years: 200 mg qds			
Cough – non-productive First line	Increase fluid intake	----------Not applicable----------			

table continues

Appendix continued

Condition	Treatment	Dosing	Likely side-effects	Significant interactions	Care needed
	Pholcodine	5–12 years: 2.5–5 mL (2.5–5 mg) qds > 12 years: 5–10 mL (5–10 mg) qds	Possible sedation	Increased sedation with alcohol, opioid analgesics, anxiolytics, hypnotics and antidepressants	Avoid in third trimester of pregnancy, liver disease Reduce dose in moderate to severe renal impairment
	Alternative second line	Simple linctus	1–12 years: 5–10 mL tds/qds (paed) > 12 years: 5–10 mL tds/qds (adult)	-------	-----None-----	
Cradle cap – see seborrhoeic dermatitis					
Cystitis	First line	Increase fluid intake	----------------Not applicable----------------		
	Second line	Any alkalinising agent	> 12 years: one sachet tds for 48 hours	Possible gastric irritation	Potassium-containing products best avoided in patients taking angiotensin-	Caution in patients with heart disease, hypertension or renal impairment

					converting enzyme inhibitors, spironolactone and potassium-sparing diuretics
Dandruff	First line	Ketoconazole (Nizoral dandruff shampoo)	All ages: apply every 3-4 days	Local irritation	----None----
	Second line	Selenium (e.g. Selsun)	> 5 years: apply twice weekly for 2 weeks then once weekly for 2 weeks	Local irritation	None, but manufacturers say avoid in first trimester of pregnancy
					None
Diarrhoea	First line	Oral rehydration therapy	Infants: 1-1½ times feed volume. Children/adults: 200–400 mL after each loose motion	----	----None----
	Second line	Loperamide	> 12 years: two stat, then one after each loose motion	Abdominal cramps, nausea and vomiting, tiredness	None
Dry eye	First line	Hypromellose	Adults: apply when needed	None	None, although manufacturers say avoid in pregnancy

table continues

Appendix continued

Condition	Treatment		Dosing	Likely side-effects	Significant interactions	Care needed
	Second line	Carbomer 940	Adults: apply tds/qds when needed	None	None, although manufacturers say avoid in pregnancy	
Dyspepsia: generalised symptoms	First line	Antacids	> 12 years: when needed after food	Possible constipation or diarrhoea dependent on metal salt used (Mg = diarrhoea, Ca and Al = constipation)	Tetracyclines, quinolones, imidazoles, phenytoin, penicillamine and bisphosphonates	Caution in patients with heart disease
	Second line	H₂ antagonists, famotidine (Pepcid AC)	> 16 years: one od (max two in 24 hours)	Diarrhoea, constipation, headache, rash	None	Manufacturers advise avoid in pregnancy/breast feeding but risk, if any, is small
	Second line	Omeprazole	>18 years: two od for 3–4 days then one od	Skin rash, GI upset	None, although manufacturers advise caution with warfarin, phenytoin and imidazoles	As H2 antagonists
Retrosternal pain (heartburn)	First line	Alginates (e.g. Gaviscon range)	> 12 years: when needed after food	None		Caution in patients with heart disease

234

Ear wax	First line	Peroxide-based products (e.g. Exterol and Otex)	> 12 years: five drops od/bd for 3–4 days	------None------
	Second line	Oil-based products (e.g. Cerumol)	All ages: five drops bd/tds	
Eczema/dermatitis	First line for maintenance	Emollients	Infant upwards: apply when needed	None, although some products contain sensitising excipients (see *BNF* section 13.1.3) ------None------
	First line for acute flare-ups	Hydrocortisone (e.g. Dermacort, Hc45, Lanacort, Zenoxone)	> 10 years: apply twice a day	------None------
	Second line for acute flare-ups	Clobetasone	> 12 years: apply twice a day	------None------
Emergency hormonal contraception	First line	Levonelle	> 16 years: two tabs immediately	Anticonvulsants, rifampicin, griseofulvin, St John's wort, ciclosporin	Conditions that might affect absorption of Levonelle, e.g. Crohn's disease	Avoid in liver disease

table continues

Appendix continued

Condition	Treatment	Dosing	Likely side-effects	Significant interactions	Care needed
Fever	First line	Paracetamol (e.g. Calpol, Disprol, Medinol)	3 months–1 year: 60–120 mg qds 1–5 years: 120–250 mg qds 6–12 years: 250–500 mg qds > 12 years: 500 mg–1 g qds	----------------None----------------	
	Alternative first line	Ibuprofen	6–12 months: 50 mg tds/qds 1–3 years: 100 mg tds 4–6 years: 150 mg tds 7–9 years: 200 mg tds 10–12 years: 300 mg tds	Gastrointestinal effects, e.g. nausea and diarrhoea	Lithium, anticoagualants, methotrexate, although children unlikely to be taking such medicines	Exercise care in asthmatics
Fungal infection	First line	Imidazoles (e.g. clotrimazole, miconazole, ketoconazole)	All ages: apply bd/tds	Burning or itching	----------None----------	
	Second line	Terbinafine (e.g. Lamisil AT)	> 16 years: apply od/bd	Itching	----------None----------	

Gingivitis	First line	Chlorhexidine gluconate (e.g. Corsodyl, Eludril)	> 12 years: 10 mL around mouth bd	Staining of teeth or tongue	----None----
Haemorrhoids	First line	Any product	> 12 years: apply bd and after each motion Perinal and Germoloids spray (>14 years) and Anusol Plus (>18 years) as contain hydrocortisone	Possible irritation	----None----
Hair loss	First line	Minoxidil (e.g. Regaine)	> 18 years: 1 mL bd	Skin irritation and rarely systemic absorption may lead to dizziness	None	Avoid in hypertension and pregnancy
Hayfever – productive generalised symptoms	First line	Allergen avoidance	----Not applicable----			
	First line medication	Loratadine	2–5 years: 5 mg (5 mL or half a tablet) od > 6 years: 10 mg (10 mL or one tablet) od	Possible sedation	None	None but manufacturers advise avoid in pregnancy

table continues

237

Appendix continued

Condition	Treatment	Dosing	Likely side-effects	Significant interactions	Care needed
	Second line medication if od dosing not controlling symptoms	Acrivastine	> 12 years: one capsule tds prn	Possible sedation	None	Avoid in moderate/severe renal impairment
Hayfever – nasal symptoms predominate	First line	Corticosteroids (e.g. beclometasone)	> 18 years: two sprays bd into each nostril. Note: fluticasone also available	Nasal irritation, bitter taste, nose bleeds	None	Avoid in glaucoma
	Second line	Antihistamine (e.g. Azelastine)	> 5 years: 1 spray bd into each nostril. Note: levocabastine also available	Nasal irritation, bitter taste	-------None-------	
Hayfever – ocular symptoms predominate	First line	Levocabastine	> 12 years: one drop bd into both eyes	Local irritation, blurred vision	-------None-------	
	Second line	Sodium cromoglicate	No lower age limit: one or two drops qds into both eyes	Local irritation, blurred vision	-------None-------	

Head lice	First line (any product due to mosaic approach to management)	Permethrin (e.g. Lyclear Crème Rinse)	> 6 months: apply to washed hair and leave on for 10 minutes	Irritation of scalp, but rare	----------None----------	
	Alternative first line	Phenothrin (e.g. Full Marks lotion)	> 6 months: Apply to dry hair and leave on for 12 hours	Irritation of scalp, but rare	None	Asthmatics should avoid alcoholic-based products As phenothrin
	Alternative first line	Malathion (e.g. Derbac-M, Prioderm)	> 6 months: Apply to dry hair and leave on for 12 hours	Irritation of scalp, but rare	None	
Inflammatory bowel syndrome	First line	Mebeverine (e.g. Colofac IBS)	> 10 years: one tablet tds	Rash, though rare	----------None----------	
	Second line	Peppermint oil (e.g. Colpermin Mintec)	> 15 years: one capsule tds	Heartburn, rarely rash	----------None----------	
Insomnia	First line	Diphenhydramine (e.g. Nytol, Dreemon)	> 16 years: 25–50 mg at night	Dry mouth, grogginess next day	Increased sedation with opioid analgesics, anxiolytics, hypnotics and antidepressants	Caution in prostate enlargement, glaucoma and liver disease

table continues

Appendix continued

Condition	Treatment	Dosing	Likely side-effects	Significant interactions	Care needed
	Second line	Promethazine (e.g. Sominex and Phenergan Nightime)	> 16 years: one tablet taken at night	Dry mouth, grogginess next day	Increased sedation with opioid analgesics, anxiolytics, hypnotics and antidepressants	Caution in prostate enlargement, glaucoma and liver disease
Malaria	First line (depends on destination)	Chloroquine (e.g. Avloclor)	Infant–13 years: mg/kg dosing 13 years: 300 mg weekly	Gastrointestinal disturbances, visual problems	Amiodarone, ciclosporin, flecainide, sotalol, terfenadine	Avoid in epilepsy
	First line (only given in combination with chloroquine)	Proguanil (e.g. Paludrine)	Infant–13 years: mg/kg dosing 13 years: 200 mg (2 tablets) od	Diarrhoea	None	Avoid in renal impairment If pregnant then folic acid 5 mg should be co-prescribed
Migraine	First line	Migraleve Pink	10–14 years: one pink tablet stat > 14 years: 2 pink tablet stat	Dry mouth, sedation, constipation	Increased sedation with opioid analgesics, anxiolytics,	Avoid in third trimester, glaucoma, prostate and

					hypnotics and antidepressants	enlargement
	Second line	Midrid	> 12 years: two stat followed by one every hour	Dizziness, rash	Monoamine oxidase inhibitors, moclobemide, beta-blockers and tricyclic antidepressants	Caution in renal and liver disease, diabetes and hypertension. Avoid in glaucoma, pregnancy and breast feeding
	Second line	Buccastem	> 18 years: one or two tablets bd	Drowsiness	Increased sedation with opioid analgesics, anxiolytics, hypnotics and antidepressants	Avoid in patients with Parkinson's disease, epilepsy, liver disease and glaucoma
Motion sickness	First line	Hyoscine (e.g. Joy-Rides)	3–4 years: half a tablet 4–7 years: one tablet 7–12 years: two tablets Note: Also available as Kwells and Junior Kwells	Dry mouth, sedation	Increased anticholinergic side-effects with tricyclic antidepressants and neuroleptics	Angle-closure glaucoma, prostate enlargement

table continues

Appendix continued

Condition	Treatment	Dosing	Likely side-effects	Significant interactions	Care needed
	Second line	Antihistamines, e.g. cinnarazine (Stugeron)	5–12 years: one tablet > 12 years: two tablets Note: a number of alternative antihistamines could be tried, e.g. cyclizine (Valoid), meclozine (Sea-Legs) and promethazine (Avomine)	Dry mouth, sedation	Increased sedation with alcohol, opioid analgesics, analgesics, anxiolytics, hypnotics and antidepressants	Angle-closure glaucoma, prostate enlargement
Mouth ulcers	First line	Choline salicylate (e.g. Bonjela, Dinnefords Teejel)	> 10 years: apply every 3–4 hours	-----------------	-----None------	
	Second line	Adcortyl or Corlan Pellets	> 12 years: apply bd–qds (Adcortyl) > 12 years: one pellet qds (Corlan)	None	None, but manufacturers state that there might be a very small risk to the human fetus in pregnancy	
Nausea and vomiting	First line for vomiting	Oral rehydration therapy	Infants: 1– 1½ times feed volume Children/adults: 200–400 mL when needed	-----------------	-----None------	

242

First line for nausea associated with gastritis	Domperidone (e.g. Motilium 10)	> 16 years: one qds after food	Rash or abdominal cramps but rare	None	None, although manufacturer advises avoidance in pregnancy
First line for nausea associated with migraine	Prochlorperazine (e.g. Buccastem)	> 18 years: one or two tablets bd	Drowsiness	Increased sedation with opioid analgesics, anxiolytics, hypnotics and antidepressants	Avoid in patients with Parkinson's disease, epilepsy, liver disease and glaucoma
Nicotine replacement therapy	See Chapter 10 (Specific product requests) for individual products				
Oral thrush	First line	Daktarin	< 2 years: 2.5 mL bd 2–6 years: 2.5 mL qds > 6 years: 5 mL qds	Nausea and vomiting	Warfarin	None

table continues

Appendix continued

Condition	Treatment		Dosing	Likely side-effects	Significant interactions	Care needed
Otitis externa	First line	Choline salicylate (e.g. Earex Plus and Audax)	> 1 year: Fill ear with drops every 3–4 hours	-----------------	----------None----------	----------None----------
	Second line	Acetic acid (e.g. Earcalm Spray)	> 12 years: one spray tds	Stinging or burning sensation		
Period pain	First line	Ibuprofen	Adults: 200–400 mg tds	Gastrointestinal effects, e.g nausea and diarrhoea Topical formulations might cause skin rash	Lithium, anticoagulants, methotrexate	Avoid in pregnancy and breast feeding, moderate/severe renal impairment and patients with a history of peptic ulcer Care in asthmatics and in mild renal impairment use lowest effective dose

						Avoid large doses in liver disease, e.g. alcoholics
PMS	Second line	Paracetamol	Adults: 500–1000 mg qds prn	None		None
	First line	Vitamin B₆	Adults: up to 100 mg od	None when given in doses for premenstrual syndrome	Levodopa when administered alone	
	Second line	Calcium	Adults: 1200 mg elemental calcium od	Nausea and flatulence	None	Caution in renal impairment
Psoriasis – plaque and scalp	First line (for flare-ups)	Coal tar (e.g. Clinitar, Exorex)	All ages: apply bd Dose might vary depending on product used	Local irritation	--------None--------	
	Second line	Emollients (for plaque psoriasis)	Birth onwards: apply prn	None, although some products contain sensitising excipients (see *BNF* section 13.1.3)	--------None--------	
Scabies	First line	Permethrin (e.g. Lyclear dermal cream)	2 months–1 year: Use up to one-eighth of a tube 1–5 years: use up to one-quarter of a tube 6–12 years: use up to half a tube > 12 years: use one full tube	Burning, stinging	--------None--------	

table continues

Appendix continued

Condition	Treatment	Dosing	Likely side-effects	Significant interactions	Care needed
	Second line	Malathion (e.g. Derbac-M, Quellada-M)	6 months–2 years: apply to whole body for 24 hours > 2 years: apply to whole body (minus head) for 24 hours	Skin irritation	------None------
Seborrhoeic dermatitis (cradle cap)	First line	Non-medicated shampoo	All ages: use on alternate days	------None------	------None------
	Second line	Dentinox Cradle Cap shampoo	All ages: apply bd during bath times		
	Second line	Coal tar (e.g. Polytar)	All age: apply bd, but will vary with product used	Local irritation	
Smoking	First line	Nicotine replacement therapy as gum, lozenges, patches, sublingual tablets and inhalator	> 18 years: Dose depends on formulation used and how heavy a smoker the patient is. See individual manufacturer literature for precise dosage instructions	Gastrointestinal disturbances	None	Patients with heart disease Avoid in pregnancy

246

| Soft tissue injuries | First line | Ibuprofen | **Systemic** > 12 years: 200–400 mg tds **Topical** > 12 years: Apply 3–4 times a day | Gastrointestinal effects, e.g nausea and diarrhoea Topical formulations might cause skin rash | Lithium, anticoagulants, methotrexate | Avoid in pregnancy and breast feeding, moderate/severe renal impairment and patients with a history of peptic ulcer Care in asthmatics and in mild renal impairment; use lowest effective dose |
| | Alternative first line | Aspirin | > 16 years: 300–900 mg every 4–6 hours | Gastrointestinal effects, e.g. nausea and diarrhoea | Anticoagulants, methotrexate | Avoid in pregnancy and breast feeding, patients with a history of peptic ulcer, severe renal impairment and liver disease Exercise care in asthmatics |

table continues

Appendix continued

Condition	Treatment	Dosing	Likely side-effects	Significant interactions	Care needed
	Second line	Paracetamol	> 12 years: 500–1000 mg qds prn	None		Avoid large doses in liver disease, e.g. alcoholics
	Second line	Rubefacients	> 5/6 years: Prn up to four times a day	Local irritation		----------None----------
Sore throat	First line	Local anaesthetics, e.g. benzocaine (Tyrozets lozenges or AAA spray)	> 3 years: one every 3 hours (Tyrozets) > 6 years: one dose every 2-3 hours prn (AAA Spray) > 12 years: two doses every 2-3 hours prn Note: other products are available that contain benzocaine and lidocaine	Can cause sensitisation reactions	None	Neonatal respiratory depression in large doses. Avoid in third trimester
	Second line	Anti-inflammatories, e.g. benzydamine (Difflam) flurbiprofen (Strefen)	> 6 years: Use every 1½–3 hours (Difflam) > 12 years: one every 3-6 hours (Strefen)	Difflam might cause stinging and tongue discoloration	None	Manufacturers of flurbiprofen state should be avoided in third trimester

				of pregnancy and advise caution in breast feeding women. Avoid in patients with peptic ulceration
Styes	First line	Warm compress		--------None--------
	Second line	Dibromopropamidine (e.g. Brolene and Golden Eye ointment)	All ages: apply tds/qds	--------None--------
			All ages: apply tds/qds (unproven benefit)	Blurred vision
Sunburn	First line	Avoidance (e.g. sunscreens)	All ages: apply tds/qds	Possible allergic reactions to sensitising agents
	Second line	Emollients	All ages: apply prn	--------None--------
Tension headache	First line	Avoid precipitating factors	--------Not applicable--------	
	Second line	Ibuprofen	Adults: 200–400 mg tds	Gastrointestinal effects, e.g nausea and diarrhoea	Lithium, anticoagulants, methotrexate Avoid in pregnancy and breast feeding,

table continues

249

Appendix continued

Condition	Treatment	Dosing	Likely side-effects	Significant interactions	Care needed
					moderate/severe renal impairment and patients with a history of peptic ulcer
					Care in asthmatics and in mild renal impairment; use lowest effective dose
	Second line	Paracetamol	Adults: 500–1000 mg qds prn	None	Avoid large doses in liver disease, e.g. alcoholics
Threadworm	First line	Mebendazole (e.g. Ovex, Pripsen Mebendazole)	> 2 years: take one tablet immediately	Abdominal pain, rash	Phenytoin and carbamazepine	Avoid in pregnancy

250

		Dosage	Side effects	Interactions	Cautions
	Second line	Piperazine (e.g. Pripsen powder or elixir)	1–6 years: one 5-ml spoonful *mane* > 6 years: one full sachet *nocte*	Diarrhoea, rash	None	Avoid in pregnancy
Vaginal thrush	First line	Imidazoles (e.g. Canesten range)	> 16 years: insert at night	Irritation	------None------	
	Second line	Fluconazole (e.g Diflucan One, Canesten Oral)	> 16 years: take immediately	Gastrointestinal disturbances	Anticoagulants, ciclosporin, rifampicin, phenytoin, tacrolimus	Avoid in pregnancy
Warts and verrucas	First line	Salicylic acid products (e.g. Compound W, Bazuka, Bazuka Extra Strength, Salactol, Salatac, Duofilm, Cuplex)	> 6 years: apply od	Local skin irritation	None	Avoid in diabetics
	Second line	Glutaraldehyde (Glutarol) or formaldehyde (Veracur)	> 12 years: apply bd	Skin irritation and staining of skin with glutaraldehyde	None	Avoid in diabetics

Index

E

F